Forensic Toxicology

Proceedings of a Symposium held at the Chemical Defence Establishment, Porton Down, 29–30 June 1972

Edited by
BRYAN BALLANTYNE
B.Sc., M.D., Ph.D., M.R.C.Path., F.I.Biol.
Senior Medical Officer (Research), Ministry of Defence

John Wright and Sons Limited
Bristol
1974

ISBN 0 7236 0356 1

Text set in 10/11 pt. IBM Press Roman, printed by photolithography, and bound in Great Britain at The Pitman Press, Bath

Dedicated to the memory
of the late
Professor Francis E. Camps

Preface

The definitions of toxicology, and attempts to divide the subject into various specialized areas, are almost as numerous as those who write about the subject. Inherent in all the definitions of toxicology is a study of the harmful effects of chemicals on biological material and an elucidation of the mechanisms of interaction of chemicals with biological systems to produce these harmful effects. When organizing this symposium on Forensic Toxicology, I had in mind as a definition of that branch of toxicology 'a specialization dealing with the legal and medical aspects of the detrimental effects of chemicals on humans'. In this symposium we were therefore concerned with the immediate and long-term consequences of accidental or deliberate poisoning, the detection of such poisoning, and with the interpretation of the possible significance of demonstrating exogenous substances in biological fluids and tissues. The latter consideration was a constant theme throughout the symposium. Thus, many substances may gain access to the body, and even be stored there, without apparently causing any ill-effects. With established toxic substances, many factors have to be considered before a cause-effect relationship can be established with any degree of certainty. The field of chemical epidemiology is clearly making many contributions which are of value to the forensic toxicologist.

Symposia are not held without considerable organisation and hard work on the part of many persons. In particular, I would like to acknowledge the help of Messrs. J. E. Bright, H. F. Colgrave, P. Coles, J. Randles, T. Webber and P. Williams. I would also like to thank the Director of the Chemical Defence Establishment for allowing us the facilities of the Establishment for the symposium.

From the staff of John Wright and Sons Ltd. I have received nothing but courtesy, patience, and help in editing these Proceedings.

BRYAN BALLANTYNE

Porton Down, Wiltshire
April 1973

Contents

Contributors

B. BALLANTYNE, B.Sc., M.D., Ph.D., M.R.C. Path., F.I.Biol.,
Medical Division, Chemical Defence Establishment, Porton Down, Wiltshire.

J. M. BARNES, C.B.E., M.B., B.Chir.,
Medical Research Council Toxicology Unit, M.R.C. Laboratories, Woodmansterne Road, Carshalton, Surrey.

A. D. BEATTIE, M.D., M.R.C.P.,
University Department of Materia Medica, Stobhill General Hospital, Glasgow.

D. J. BLACKMORE, M.B.E., M.Phil., M.I.Biol.,
Department of Aviation and Forensic Pathology, R.A.F. Institute of Pathology and Tropical Medicine, Halton, Buckinghamshire: attached to Home Office Central Research Establishment, Aldermaston, Reading, Berkshire. Present address: Equine Research Station, Balaton Lodge, Newmarket, Suffolk.

R. W. BRIMBLECOMBE, Ph.D., D.Sc., F.I.Biol.,
Medical Division, Chemical Defence Establishment, Porton Down, Wiltshire. Present address: The Research Institute, Smith, Kline and French Laboratories, Welwyn Garden City, Herts.

P. LESLEY BIDSTRUP, M.D., F.R.C.P., F.R.A.C.P.,
Formerly, Department for Research in Industrial Medicine (MRC), The London Hospital.

The late Professor F. E. CAMPS, M.D., F.R.C.P., F.R.C.Path., D.M.J., D.T.M. & H.

E. G. C. CLARKE, M.A., Ph.D., D.Sc., F.R.I.C.,
Department of Physiology, The Royal Veterinary College, London.

A. S. CURRY, M.A., Ph.D., F.R.I.C., F.R.C.Path.,
Home Office Central Research Establishment, Aldermaston, Reading, Berkshire.

R. A. DALLEY, F.R.I.C., F.I.F.S.T.,
City Analyst's Department, Leeds, Yorkshire.

K. FLETCHER, B.A., Ph.D.,
Industrial Hygiene Research Laboratory, Imperial Chemical Industries Ltd., Alderley Park, Nr. Macclesfield, Cheshire.

D. J. GEE, M.B., B.S., M.R.C.Path., D.M.J.,
Department of Forensic Medicine, School of Medicine, University of Leeds, Yorkshire.

M. A. GREEN, M.B., Ch.B., D.Obst., R.C.O.G., D.C.H., D.M.J.,
Department of Forensic Medicine, School of Medicine, University of Leeds, Yorkshire.

A. C. MOFFAT, B.Pharm., Ph.D., A.R.I.C., M.P.S.,
Home Office Central Research Establishment, Aldermaston, Reading, Berkshire.

L. A. PERKIN, B.Sc., Ll.B., F.R.I.C., F.I.F.S.T.,
City Analyst's Department, Leeds, Yorkshire.

ANN E. ROBINSON, B.Pharm., Ph.D., F.R.I.C.,
Department of Forensic Medicine, The London Hospital Medical College, University of London.

M. H. P. SAYERS, O.B.E., M.D., F.R.C.Path.,
Medical Services Division, Department of Employment, London.

Methodology and Interpretation in Forensic Toxicology

A. S. CURRY
Home Office Central Research Establishment, Aldermaston, Berkshire

Methodology and interpretation are but a relatively small part of an investigation into a sudden death for which no cause can be found or in which suspicious circumstances indicate that poison may be involved. The beginning of the chain of events is with the general practitioner, hospital physician, pathologist or police officer who finds himself with a body for which paperwork has to be completed. If his suspicions are not aroused then the case will never arrive at the forensic science laboratory.

In a recent case in which a husband was convicted of murder, the general practitioner had the courage to withdraw his death certificate which stated that the deceased had died of natural causes. In the Barlow case involving a murderous injection of insulin the detective sergeant, called in to 'rubber stamp' the drowning of a wife in the bath, noticed that the circumstances did not agree with the story that the husband told and he started a full criminal investigation; photographs were taken and senior officers, together with the Home Office pathologist and laboratory staff, started enquiring into an apparently straightforward death. The sergeant's vigilance, like that of the general practitioner's, was amply rewarded. I would, therefore, at the beginning of a paper dealing with forensic toxicology like to stress that it is only by good police work that an investigation into murder will succeed. The medical and laboratory expertise may provide a satisfactory explanation for the cause of death, but circumstantial evidence is very rarely enough to prove a murder. What is needed is a very good police investigation that will show that circumstances are not what they appear to be and that one of the witnesses is lying. I well remember the comment in one police division where it was said that a policewoman was sent to interview the relatives in all cases of sudden death because she was extremely sympathetic. My only comment was that I hoped she had been on a C.I.D. course.

The next link in the chain is the pathologist who has to take samples for the analysis. It is impossible to over-emphasize the importance of his work. I have experience of cases in which if the pathologist had not tied off the stomach and the upper small intestine at one-foot intervals before they were transported in the bottom of a glass jar 50 miles by road, the required interpretation of when the deceased had taken the poison, or had been given it, would have been impossible. Knowledge of the area of diffusion around injection sites, realization that one drop of urine may be vital, the need for lungs, brain and/or spleen in particular cases – all these emphasize the very high degree of specialized knowledge that the forensic pathologist must have. I well remember the first case in which I was asked to perform toxicological analyses: the police officer arrived at the Laboratory, having travelled 20 miles by bus with a bucket containing, mixed together, the main organs of the deceased. The situation was not improved by the information that the coroner was going on holiday in a week's time and perhaps he could have a written report by then!

We are now at the stage when the organs have arrived at the laboratory. It is of interest to note that in 1970 nearly 2000 cases of toxicological investigations were done in the forensic science service. Two types of cases arrive; firstly, those in which confirmation is needed that a suicide note saying that the person has taken 5 g. of cyanide and 120 Seconal tablets is in fact authentic. The second case, which is apparently more challenging, concerns those in which a note arrives 'query poison– no cause of death'. I would like to postulate that in fact both cases should be treated very similarly, because it has been my experience that the most interesting cases are those in which the circumstantial evidence is not borne out by the analyses. In such cases, when there is a suicide note or it is apparently a case of accidental poisoning in a child, and the analytical results do not bear out the circumstantial evidence, it is often with trepidation that the toxicologist has to turn to his police colleagues and say 'I'm sorry I just do not believe what you have told me'. That this situation arises bears out the fact that the United Kingdom has a very good 'watchdog' organization for the detection of homicidal poisoning. It is not a perfect system, but in this paper I hope to indicate some of the difficulties that present themselves to the investigators, be they police, pathologists or toxicologists, and by showing the problems perhaps point the way in which research can help to answer them.

Let me now try to discuss methodology and interpretation of results within the context of forensic toxicology. I see the toxicologist's role as that of finding any abnormal chemical that may have been taken into the system and of being able to indicate, to the pathologist, normality from abnormality. The death certificate cannot be signed by the toxicologist, but as in all branches of chemical pathology, the pathologist will lean heavily on his chemist colleague.

As fas as methodology is concerned, it has been a cardinal principle in the shaping of my professional expertise to base the analysis completely on a chemical approach. The facial paralysis coupled with the beginning of convulsions in a patient who has undergone surgery for hyperparathyroidism may indeed be due to hypocalcaemia but equally well it may be the result of phenothiazine side-effect or, indeed, administration of strychnine by his wife. The pipe leading from a car exhaust to within three inches of the face of a dead man in his car could rightly lead to the conclusion that the deceased died of carbon monoxide poisoning, but unless analyses for hypnotics are performed who is to say that he was not unconscious in the car before the pipe was connected? In one such apparently simple case in which I was involved, there was only 3 per cent of carbon monoxide in the blood. I therefore come to my first main point – that is, as many analyses as possible should be performed in each and every case, notwithstanding the circumstances.

In order to discuss methodology it is first necessary to consider the different chemical classifications of poisons that may be present in the deceased. This symposium, by its papers, indicates the wide classifications that are available. We have gaseous poisons, such as carbon monoxide, volatile poisons such as cyanide, the metallic poisons of mercury and lead, organic poisons ranging from the barbiturates, methadone, and morphine, to the quaternary ammonium compounds including paraquat, as well as tests designed to show that the normal metabolism of the body has been interfered with by such poisons as cholinesterase inhibitors and monoamine oxidase inhibitors.

In each individual case the toxicological analyses have to be considered as an operational research problem. The absorption through skin of an organophosphorus compound or the acute ingestion of barbiturate will both finish up as a series of jars on the toxicologist's bench. He will sit and look at them and wonder what he can best do in the time available. Only by a systematic analysis can the full truth emerge. In addition to his chemical tests he has to have a clear knowledge of the concentrations that are likely to be found in different organs. There are about as many variants of the practical approach as there are authors, and in this paper I can only reflect my own approach to the problem. Depending on the circumstances of the death, the contents of the alimentary tract, the liver, and the brain are probably the best approach for searching for volatile poisons. Nowadays with the advent of 'head-space' analysis using gas chromatography the problem of volatiles has been largely overcome. In this context can also be included the volatile gases, but clearly there is a wide area of research to be covered as far as 'normal' gases are concerned. The problems associated with anaesthesia and inhalation for anoxic experiences are probably best tackled this way, but this is a generalization that must depend on each individual case. The possibility that the death on the operating table is from a combination of contaminated nitrous oxide in a phenacetin addict who was fed two days beforehand by an enthusiastic friend collecting wild mushrooms has to be faced. The fact that the patient is a farmer who has been involved in spraying crops or taking tranquillizers prescribed by his doctor as well as drinking lead-contaminated water from his garden well, may add to the problem. All aspects have to be investigated. The number of volatile poisons is very large indeed ranging from cyanide, the alcohols, halogenated hydrocarbons such as carbon tetrachloride, chloroform, and the dry-cleaning agents, to yellow phosphorus. To continue this systematic chemical search, the metallic poisons have to be considered. Perhaps lead, thallium, and arsenic together with mercury take pride of place, but every element must be considered; beryllium, thorotrast, and cadmium are poisons which would probably not always cross the mind of the physician investigating a patient who is ill. The methodology concerned with such cases varies tremendously: the diagnosis of thallium poisoning may be made from a single hair from the deposits at the root seen under a microscope, but for arsenic an atomic reactor may be necessary. It seems likely that flameless atomic absorption spectrophotometry will be the method of choice in the future and at the Central Research Establishment we are, I think, pioneering work into multi-element lamps which, hopefully, will be useful in this area. The inorganic field concerns not only metals but ions such as fluoride and chlorate as well as those bizarre situations when patients receive drips which are not what they are supposed to be. In one case in which I was involved a sudden onset of a gastro-intestinal disorder in a mental patient was found to be due to fluoride poisoning and was only discovered by systematic analysis. If routine tests for the presence of anionic poisons had not been conducted, it is extremely likely that this case would never have been unravelled. It is a natural reaction to think in terms of metallic or poisonous plant poisoning in such cases, but the less obvious must not be forgotten. They must be incorporated into a routine screen. Cases involving anions are fairly frequent. Bromide may be coupled with paraldehyde and tranquillizers or even, indeed, with lithium in patients in mental hospitals. These are other examples of the chemically bizarre situations in which one is asked to look for digoxin, tranquillizer (unnamed), antidiabetic drug with a *soupçon* of barbiturates, bromide, or perhaps alcohol.

The poisons that are soluble in organic solvents from different *p*H's of the tissues make up well over 2000 in number. They range from strongly acidics such as salicylic acid and the phenoxyacetic acids to the weakly acidic drugs such as barbiturates and Doriden, through neutral drugs such as meprobamate, to the bases, which are the compounds that are soluble in organic solvent from aqueous alkaline solution and which can be as divergent as nicotine, strychnine, and Librium. The quaternary ammonium compounds such as succinylcholine and tubocurarine must not be forgotten. Most of the techniques for the analyses of these drugs are relatively straightforward, involving an isolation stage followed by purification using either paper, thin layer or gas chromatography, with a subsequent identification stage. This latter stage can be relatively unspecific when a general chromatogenic spray is used, or there may be an immediate specific stage in which derivatives are formed indicating functional groups on the molecule. Indeed, such techniques may lead to the conclusion that a specific identification has been achieved. Identification can also follow the use of infra-red spectroscopy or mass spectrometry and there is no doubt that these latter two techniques are becoming *sine qua non* for the toxicological laboratory.

Unfortunately the toxicologist is not complete in his investigations when he has considered the volatiles, the inorganics, and the extractable organics, albeit that these latter include the quaternary ammonium compounds. The latter category can be extracted by the formation of ion pairs and the Home Office Central Research Establishment has produced methods for the detection and estimation of what were considered to be undetectable drugs such as tubocurarine and succinylcholine. The pattern of toxicology is nowhere better typified than in the Coppolino case where it was alleged that Dr. Coppolino had injected his wife with succinylcholine. Surely the need for research in toxicology is kept acutely alive by such cases, where poisons which were previously thought to be undetectable are presented to the toxicologist. It is well known that Barlow believed that insulin was undetectable. It is a continuing challenge to the toxicologist to be aware of such cases so that, although one person may achieve his ambition of murdering his wife, or two, or three, another husband does not. In addition to the various categories of poisons I have mentioned must not be forgotten the difficult poisons such as digoxin. Radioimmunoassays have only recently been introduced in forensic toxicology but already methods have been developed at the Central Research Establishment for the quantitative measurement of post-mortem insulin and digoxin levels.

The subject of this paper is half devoted to methodology in forensic toxicology, but by mentioning radioimmunoassays I have skipped over a century of analytical methodology. It goes without saying that I believe that in forensic toxicology, and I exclude clinical toxicology entirely from this, the laboratory should be equipped with every type of analytical apparatus. This will naturally involve machines for extraction procedures which we at the Central Research Establishment are concerned with, automating from the 100 g. of liver to the 4 ml. of urine scale, as well as automatic evaporation devices. Apparatus for chromatographic operations followed by ultra-violet, visible, and infra-red spectrographic analyses, coupled with enzyme tests, mass spectrometry, and microscopes for the localization of drugs in individual cells are all needed. By saying this I am automatically implying that it is not possible for the small laboratory without access to specialized analytical procedures to undertake a full toxicological examination. Some of you will immediately think that this is not possible in all countries. I would entirely agree with you but point out that somewhere along the line somebody should indicate the ideal situation.

We have discussed in detail the various types of poisons that may be encountered in toxicological investigations – volatiles, metals, anions, organic quaternary ammonium compounds, the difficult poisons like insulin and digoxin – but we must not forget the plant poisons like *Amanita phalloides*. Another most difficult case is that in which a young child is found to have a yellow liver with complete fat infiltration. This may be due to yellow phosphorus, sulphate, *Amanita phalloides*, or 'Reye's syndrome', which, as far as we know, is a genuine pathological condition not involving poison but strongly suggestive of it. The methodology used in investigations of these varieties of poisons that may be encountered varies tremendously; in the interpretation of results, however, a full consideration has to be taken of the method of analyses. Two examples will serve to show the care that is necessary. For many years ammonium sulphate precipitation of protein was used before extracting the filtrate for barbiturate. It has now been shown that this is a highly inefficient method in that less than 5 per cent total barbiturate may be extracted from the protein-free filtrate; one reads therefore of cases in which 'no barbiturate was found', but in fact it may well have been that the liver or other tissue contained tens of milligrams of barbiturate in one hundred grammes of tissue, but it was not found because of deficiencies in the analysis. Similarly, if one is looking for fluoride in a dialysate it is absolutely vital to make sure that the dialysis fluid is acid, otherwise formation of insoluble calcium fluoride may prevent the ion appearing in the dialysing fluid. The yield must be clearly assessed before the interpretation can begin and we are fortunate that in toxicological analysis the fatal dose often exceeds the therapeutic or 'normal' level by at least a factor of ten. The decomposition of a liver yielding perhaps 30 per cent more barbiturate in the decomposed than in the fresh sample is of relatively little significance, although this may affect conclusions concerning the time that occurred between ingestion and death. In lead poisoning, however, it will be emphasized later in these Proceedings that not only must the lead level be measured in blood, but also the haemoglobin content. I wonder if it is sufficiently realized that, in the diffusion of alcohol from blood, the blood must be deproteinized before diffusion is attempted; if this is not done the solid matrix after diffusion will still contain alcohol and the result reported by the analyst will certainly be very low indeed compared to the true value.

We are, therefore, at the stage where the analyst has got to consider a very large number of drugs. He must know the methods that must be employed to give results that are interpretable. He has to know the yields that can be expected, and most important he must know that his techniques are capable of detecting therapeutic, or at least subtoxic, levels of drugs that he may encounter. He has yet another problem, and that is the ability of the body at post mortem to be a most efficient chemical factory. He must know that alcohol, cyanide, and a host of amines can be produced as post-mortem artefacts. There will be few scientists who would hesitate to say that tens of milligrams per one hundred ml. of cyanide in blood constituted a lethal level, but only in the last few years has it been realized that cyanide, that most simple molecule, is produced in such amounts as a post-mortem artefact; it does not come entirely from thiocyanate and clearly a tremendous amount of research has to be done if the forensic toxicologist is to be even more certain of his interpretations in cases of suspected cyanide poisoning. The distribution of drugs in the organs is another vital factor when one is trying to interpret results. The increased concentration of cyanide in the spleen, or barbiturates in the liver, or glutethimide and morphine in the bile are typical examples, but the high concentration of many drugs in the urine is also of great importance. The validity of urine analyses in relation to alcohol, and the concentration effects, particularly, for example, with morphine, make this the ideal and universally easily collectable fluid. The use of urine to show the presence of a drug is, in my opinion, of paramount importance.

I have mentioned so many wide classifications of poisons that it is perfectly obvious that the analyses cannot be completed in a day or two and indeed that sophisticated instrumentation is necessary if a complete analysis for all poisons is to be efficient. It is equally obvious that the analyses must be directed to those organs in which the poisons are most likely to concentrate, and therefore that the forensic pathologist must know a tremendous amount about the problems facing the forensic toxicologist. This is a point that I cannot too highly stress. I am strongly of the opinion that if an efficient investigation is to proceed there must be the closest collaboration between the pathologist and the toxicologist. Even the container that is used for the organs must receive full consideration. I do not yet know of a better alternative to glass, albeit that it is inconvenient to the pathologist because of its weight.

In many investigations a specific analysis is requested and it behoves the toxicologist, therefore, to be able to look at the literature and choose the method most suitable for a specific drug. I recently did a survey of 5000 references since 1966 on the aetiology, methodology, and interpretation of results for poisons, and published 1500 references in a book. This involved a vast amount of labour and clearly the collection, annotation, filing, and indexing of data, both as far as analytical methodology and the interpretation of results are concerned, is of paramount importance to the toxicologist. Interpretation comes from comparison with similar cases. At the Home Office Central Research Establishment we have been in the data-collecting industry for the last six years and have studied this problem in depth. Two problems became apparent. First, there is the problem of collecting, collating, and indexing analytical data so that if in an analysis a particular ultra-violet, infra-red, or chromatographic parameter is obtained, it is possible to search the collection to see if the data matches that of a particular known substance or substances. This involves the transference of analogue information to digital form and the transference of that data to a computer system. Secondly, as far as the general literature related to methodology and interpretation is concerned, it is necessary to search about 2000 journals every two weeks and then to index, after collection, the papers that concern the toxicologist. As I see it at the moment, we have succeeded in organizing this collection of data at the Central Research Establishment and in addition have collected a comprehensive register of human toxicology in which all analytical results of fatal cases, known to the Forensic Science Service, are collated at the Central Research Establishment. This includes the results known to INFORM and to the International Association of Forensic Toxicologists.

We found our greatest problem was in the area of indexing and indeed in keeping an index up to date. The solution has been found to be in the use of a computer. At the present time we are on a Burroughs time-shared computer at Brussels, because our data formed the basis for an exercise in computing for the Police National Computer. Leo Kazyak, from the U.S.A., has been on a Research Fellowship at the Central Research Establishment for a year, and has demonstrated the viability of such a system. He is at the present time concerned with transferring the data to our own 'in-house' computer – a Hewlett Packard 2100. The basis of the system is that every item of data is described in terms of 'key words'. An infra-red spectrum, for example, can be described in a series of six or seven digital numbers corresponding to the major peaks of the spectrum. If a scientific paper is required to be indexed it can be described in a series of key words; usually about ten words are sufficient to describe a paper fully. In the early stages, it was recognized that a dictionary of reliable key words was required and a great deal of effort went into preparing and testing the efficiency of a key-word thesaurus. Once this had been done it was necessary to convert scientific papers into the jargon of the computer, that is to say, convert each abstract or indeed the full paper into a series of key words and allocate each paper a consecutive number. Now that over 10,000 papers have been placed in the store of the computer, it is only necessary for us to dial the Brussels computer and insert the words in which we are interested – for example, *methaqualone, ident, level*; in this way, any papers concerned with the identification of methaqualone and its level in tissue will be returned to us in seconds as a series of numbers corresponding to the original papers. For storage purposes all papers have been microfilmed and are being supplied to the regional forensic science laboratories. It is possible in this way to keep completely up to date, day by day, and so avoid the problems associated with multi-factor searching – for example, where does one file a paper concerned with the atomic absorption spectrophotometry of lead coupled with its measurement by mass spectrometry and colorimetric measurements in blood, urine, brain, kidney, and liver? The paper may also include details of pathological and clinical conditions and, indeed, discuss not only lead but also copper, arsenic, cadmium, and zinc. The problems of indexing such a paper are completely overcome by the computer because one can feed all these key words into it and hence there is one record rather than perhaps ten reprints lingering in ten different files.

The problem of data retrieval is going to become exponentially more difficult as the years go by. There is at the present time no central data collecting agency on an international scale, and we find enthusiastic information centres all collecting their relatively small data banks. The value of co-operation between such banks at the Chemical Defence Establishment and the Central Research Establishment has become obvious to us, as there is such a small distance between the two organizations, but the registers of human toxicology prepared by Eckert in the States and the attempts of such a system by the California Association of Criminalists under Brian Finkle have shown that a much more co-ordinated system is needed. Leo Kazyak, under the auspices of the International Association of Forensic Toxicologists, is trying to do just this. We require compatible computer systems and a means for checking that papers recognized in the literature as being important by ten different experts are not coded ten times but only once; the variabilities of machines used for analyses must be catered for, and as I hope I have indicated in this paper the vagaries of different isolation and quantitative procedures must be taken into account before a true interpretation is arrived at.

The problems of interpretation are indeed manifest: we have all been perfectly capable persons with a blood alcohol of 300 mg. per 100 ml. and have sent people to hospital in a state of severe alcoholic intoxication with blood levels of 100 mg. per 100 ml. My own concern with this problem has been dramatized by the discovery of a person with 30 mg. per 100 ml. of butobarbitone in the blood being in a 'normal' condition. The future, I am sure, lies in the discovery of the biochemical lesions that occur in poisoning. This is an aspect in which the Home Office Central Research Establishment is intimately concerned, for after all it is not sufficient to merely discover the poison or drug – we must eventually be able to show that it is having an effect.

The Use of Enzymes in the Detection of Drugs

A. C. MOFFAT
Home Office Central Research Establishment, Aldermaston, Berkshire

Before discussing the ways in which enzymes may be used in the analysis of drugs, it might be of interest to note that there are 15 enzymes in use as therapeutic agents as listed in the *Extra Pharmacopoeia* (1967) (*Table* 1). Of these, hyaluronidase

Table 1. Enzymes in use as therapeutic agents (from *Extra Pharmacopoeia* (1967)).

Alpha Amylase	Penicillinase
Bromelains	Pepsin
Chymotrypsin	Plasmin
Deoxyribonuclease	Streptodornase
Diastase	Streptokinase
Hyaluronidase	Trypsin
Pancreatin	Urokinase
Papain	

and pancreatin both appear in the *British Pharmacopoeia* (1968), which gives assays to measure the activity of the enzyme preparations. In the case of hyaluronidase, the assay is carried out by comparison with a standard preparation. However, the vast majority of drugs are much simpler organic molecules and the bulk of this paper is concerned with their detection, identification, and quantitation.

In a simple enzyme reaction (*Fig.* 1) the apoenzyme combines first with a

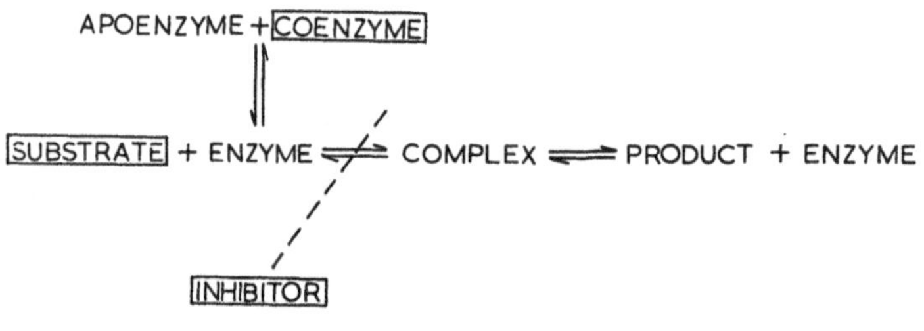

Fig. 1. A simple enzyme reaction.

coenzyme (cofactor) to form a holoenzyme which combines further with the substrate to form a complex. This later splits to give the product, or products, together with the original holoenzyme. A reaction of this type may therefore be used to detect a drug if it is:

A. A naturally occurring coenzyme or could be used as an activator of the enzyme,
B. A substrate for the enzyme, or
C. An inhibitor, whether competitive or non-competitive.

There are over 200 different enzymes available (Guilbault, 1970) and they can be used as normal laboratory reagents provided that their conditions of storage and use are optimized. They are best stored as dried powders rather than solutions, although solutions may remain stable for many weeks when refrigerated. Factors to be optimized in the reaction medium are the *p*H, temperature, salt concentration, absence of heavy metal ions which might otherwise act as inhibitors, and concentration of the appropriate coenzyme. To be of use the enzyme should be obtained in the crystallized form, or at least in a pure state, it should be as cheap as possible, easily available, and preferably have the same activity from batch to batch. Enzymes are usually sold in units (one unit of any enzyme is that amount which will catalyse the transformation of one micromole of any substrate per minute under defined conditions) or in mg. with a stated specific activity (number of units of enzyme activity per unit of protein; usually given as units/mg. protein).

A. METHODS USING THE DRUG AS AN ACTIVATOR

There are three types of activators of enzymatic reactions:

(*a*) Kinases which convert the inactive form of the enzyme (zymogen) into an active form, e.g. streptokinase;

(*b*) Coenzymes, which are mostly nucleotides;

(*c*) Miscellaneous activators such as Mg^{++} and compounds containing sulphydryl groups.

For obvious reasons there are very few examples of drugs acting in enzymatic reactions in this way, but the method of use can be illustrated by an assay for pyridoxal phosphate (vitamin B_6) in blood (Maruyama and Coursin, 1968). The reactions are:

$$\begin{matrix}\text{Tyrosine} \\ \text{apodecarboxylase}\end{matrix} + \begin{matrix}\text{Pyridoxal} \\ \text{phosphate}\end{matrix} \longrightarrow \begin{matrix}\text{Tyrosine} \\ \text{holodecarboxylase}\end{matrix}$$

$$\text{Tyrosine-1-}^{14}\text{C} \xrightarrow{\text{Holoenzyme}} \text{Tyramine} + {}^{14}CO_2$$

Excess tyrosine apodecarboxylase (from *Streptococcus faecalis*) is mixed with known amounts of pyridoxal phosphate to form the holoenzyme. This is then used to decarboxylate the substrate (tyrosine) and the rate of the reaction is followed by the decrease in radioactivity of the incubation medium due to the loss of ^{14}C-carbon dioxide. Controls, without the pyridoxal phosphate, are also run and the results are used to construct a standard curve. Extracts of brain, blood, and liver can then be analysed using the curve.

Some peptidases have enhanced activity in the presence of compounds containing sulphydryl groups because they remove traces of heavy metals which would otherwise be inhibitory (Bell, Davidson, and Scarborough, 1961). Thus, it might be possible to assay 6-mercaptopurine, methimazole, and other drugs containing sulphydryl groups in this way.

B. METHODS USING THE DRUG AS THE SUBSTRATE

Probably the most well known example of the use of this method is the assay of ethanol using alcohol dehydrogenase (ADH).

$$C_2H_5OH + NAD^+ \underset{}{\overset{ADH}{\rightleftharpoons}} CH_3CHO + NADH + H^+$$

$$CH_3CHO \xrightarrow{NH_2CONHNH_2} NH_2CONHNCHCH_3$$

The dehydrogenation of ethanol to acetaldehyde involves the reduction of NAD (nicotinamide-adenine dinucleotide, also known as DPN, diphosphopyridine nucleotide, and coenzyme I) to NADH. Since the enzyme acts as a catalyst and only speeds the attainment of equilibrium, the reaction must be forced to completion by trapping the product, in this case by the use of semicarbazide. The *Catalytic Constant* of an enzyme is the number of moles of substrate acted on per minute by one mole of enzyme, and it is of interest to note that values up to 5,000,000 can be obtained for some enzymes. However, even though an enzyme has a large catalytic constant, sufficient enzyme should always be used to ensure a rapid assay in case any inhibitors are present. An excess of the coenzyme must always be present because it is consumed during the reaction.

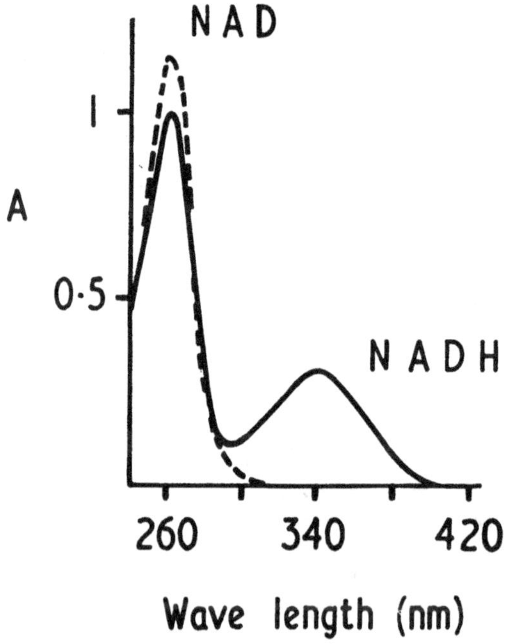

Fig. 2. The ultra-violet absorption spectrum of nicotinamide-adenine dinucleotide (NAD; dotted line) and its reduced form, NADH (continuous line).

The reaction may be studied (*a*) by measuring the total change that has taken place, or (*b*) by a kinetic method. In general the latter is quicker since one does not have to wait for the reaction to go to completion or to reach equilibrium. The accuracy and precision of both methods are comparable and are about 1 per cent (Guilbault, 1968). In both cases a standard curve is prepared with samples of known alcohol concentration. The course of the reaction is measured by the loss of the substrate (ethanol), the formation of the product (acetaldehyde) or the conversion of the coenzyme NAD to NADH.

It can be seen from *Fig.* 2 that the absorbance of NADH at 340 nm. and the lack of absorbance of NAD at this wavelength allows easy measurement of any dehydrogenase system. The nucleotide NADP (nicotinamide-adenine dinucleotide phosphate, also known as TPN, triphosphopyridinenucleotide, and coenzyme II) and the reduced form (NADPH) can be measured similarly. The ultra-violet method of measurement is the one generally used and has been modified in automated methods for the estimation of blood alcohol levels (e.g. Goldberg and Rydberg, 1965). Greater sensitivity of detection may be obtained using fluorescent methods, which are discussed later.

To be able to estimate either the substrate or the product they must be capable of being measured easily and separately in the presence of one another. The actual method depends upon the nature of the enzymatic reaction, i.e. whether the enzyme is an oxidase, decarboxylase, esterase, etc. *Table 2* is a list of those drugs for which

Table 2. Enzymatic methods of drug analysis using the drug as the substrate

Drug	*Tissue*	*Enzyme*	*Reference*
Ethanol	Blood	Alcohol dehydrogenase	Bonnichsen (1965) Jones *et al.* (1970)
Ethanol		Alcohol oxidase	Guilbault and Sadar (1969a)
Paraldehyde	Serum and C.S.F.	Alcohol dehydrogenase	Thurston *et al.* (1968)
Oxalic Acid	Plasma and urine	Oxalic acid decarboxylase	Crawhall and Watts (1961) Mayer *et al.* (1963) Ribeiro and Elliot (1964)
Hyoscyamine		L-Hyoscyamine-acyl-hydrolase	Seiler and Werner (1965)
Pethidine		Pethidine esterase	Ammon and Kamphues (1969)
20-Ketosteroids	Plasma	20-β-Hydroxysteroid dehydrogenase	Hübener (1965)

enzymatic methods of analysis are available and where the drug acts as the substrate for the reaction. Either alcohol dehydrogenase or alcohol oxidase can be used for ethanol, each with a different specificity for substrates. Alcohol dehydrogenase (from yeast) is most sensitive to ethyl alcohol whereas alcohol oxidase (from a fungus) is most sensitive to methyl alcohol, so giving a method of estimating a mixture of the two. Paraldehyde can be depolymerized by dilute acid to its monomer and then estimated by the alcohol dehydrogenase system by measuring the decrease in NADH as the acetaldehyde is reduced to ethanol. Ketosteroids in plasma can also be assayed by a dehydrogenase system. Manometric measurements, using a Warburg apparatus, have been used to determine oxalate in plasma and urine by measuring the amount of carbon dioxide formed using oxalic acid decarboxylase. In the case of hyoscyamine, the amount of acid formed by hydrolysis was measured by titrating with sodium hydroxide solution. Other techniques that can be used to monitor enzymatic reactions include polarography, potentiometric titrations, colour measurement, and radiochemical methods.

One way of using cholinesterase came our way recently (Stevens, H. M., and Moffat, A. C., unpublished observations). We had difficulty in identifying succinylcholine in urine after the administration of an intravenous dose. The usual methods of instrumental analyses were unsuitable because of the aliphatic and quaternary nature of the compound. Therefore, thin-layer chromatography was used and two solvent systems using two spray reagents were developed. That the compound was a choline ester was shown by running two urine extracts on a plate, spraying one with a solution of cholinesterase in phosphate buffer (*p*H 8·0) and the other with buffer alone, and incubating the plate in a moisture tank for an hour at 37°C. After spraying with iodoplatinate reagent the spot previously sprayed with buffer solution was visible whilst that sprayed with the enzyme was not.

Enzymes come from a variety of different sources: alcohol dehydrogenase from yeast, alcohol oxidase from a fungus of the Polyporoceae family, oxalic acid decarboxylase from the wood-rot fungus *Collybia velutipes,* pethidine esterase from rabbit liver, and 20-ketosteroid dehydrogenase from *Streptomyces hydrogenans.* It is obvious that for every drug that is assayed a suitable specific enzyme must be available. The few reported methods of analysis using such enzymes show how difficult it is to obtain them. Liver microsomes or serum may contain some enzymes that metabolize specific drugs, but a lot of research would be needed before the appropriate enzymes could be isolated and characterized. One method that might produce an enzyme using a single drug as substrate is being considered at the Microbiological Research Establishment (Wade, 1972). A continuous culture, containing a number of species of bacteria, is fed with a drug; one strain takes over the colony and hopefully includes the drug into its metabolism. The bacteria could then be harvested and the enzyme responsible for the degradation of the drug isolated.

Once we have a specific enzyme for a drug, many quick ways of drug detection and estimation can be produced. There are three main ways in which I think developments could go.

The first would be to use the enzyme to confer specificity to what is essentially a non-specific chemical method. For example, if a drug is extracted from a biological material and then examined by fluorescence spectroscopy, although the sensitivity is good, the background might be so high as to make an identification from the emission spectrum impossible. However, if the spectrum was obtained and an appropriate enzyme then introduced to convert the drug to a non-fluorescent compound, the difference spectrum obtained before and after the addition of the enzyme would represent the spectrum of the drug itself.

The second would be to make testing 'sticks' similar to those already available for biochemical tests in urine. For example, Clinistix (Ames Company) are used to detect glucose in urine. They are sticks impregnated with glucose oxidase, peroxidase, *o*-tolidine, and a red dye. When dipped into a solution containing glucose the glucose oxidase converts the glucose to gluconic acid with the production of hydrogen peroxide. This, together with the peroxidase, then converts the *o*-tolidine to a blue compound which, with the red dye, gives a purple colour; i.e. a positive reaction. (This is an example of the use of a coupled reaction – the formation of the product(s) of the second reaction being used to monitor the progress of the first reaction.) The sensitivity of the test is in the region of 10–100 mg. per cent provided that there are no inhibitors present in the urine. If a series of enzymes could be obtained for drugs a whole new area of quick but specific drug identification could be opened.

The third way in which drug metabolizing enzymes might be used is by utilizing an insolubilized form of the enzyme. In the past a major objection to the use of enzymes as reagents has been their high cost. If they could be recovered after a test, it would cut the cost of an analysis tremendously. Enzites (Miles-Seravac) are enzymes covalently bonded on to water insoluble supports such as carboxymethyl-cellulose or agarose gel. The Enzite comes as a freeze-dried powder which could be used in batch methods of analysis. It could be used, then filtered, washed, and dried, to recover the enzyme. Or a column could be used, in a continuous method of analysis; ethanol estimations, for example, could be done this way. Perhaps the most exciting aspect would be the manufacture of a drug-specific electrode.

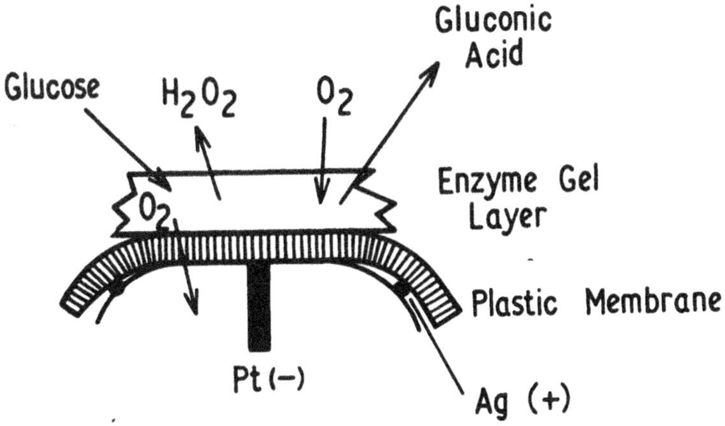

Fig. 3. A glucose-specific electrode.

Fig. 3 shows a glucose-specific electrode. It is in fact an oxygen electrode with an enzyme gel layer held on by a nylon mesh to the outside of the membrane surrounding the electrode. Without glucose present in the solution to be measured, oxygen diffuses through the enzyme layer and plastic membrane and is reduced on the platinum cathode to give a response. If the electrode is then placed in a glucose solution, the glucose diffuses into the enzyme layer, uses oxygen which would otherwise have reached the cathode, and therefore causes a reduced reading of the electrode. When there is excess oxygen present and the glucose concentration is below the K_m of the insolubilized enzyme, the reduction in current is linear with respect to the glucose concentration.

Both oxidase and deaminase reactions can be used in specific electrodes (which would measure the production of O_2 and NH_4^+ respectively). It goes without saying that if a series of similar electrodes could be prepared for drug analyses, they would be very useful indeed.

C. METHODS USING THE DRUG AS AN INHIBITOR

There are many drugs on the market which are enzyme inhibitors and a list of the main groups together with some examples is given below:

1. Monoamine oxidase inhibitors: tranylcypromine, phenelzine, nialamide (antidepressants).
2. Carbonic anhydrase inhibitors: acetazolamide (diuretic).
3. Cholinesterase inhibitors: neostigmine, physostigmine, di-*iso*propylflurophosphate (all used for the treatment of glaucoma).
4. Xanthine oxidase inhibitors: allopurinol (used for the treatment of gout).
5. Anticoagulants: heparin (an antithrombin).
6. Phosphodiesterase inhibitors: these may be used in the future as antidepressants or bronchodilators.
7. Chemotherapeutic agents: sulphonamides (the principle of blocking a biochemical reaction by the use of a compound similar to the usual substrate is the basis of chemotherapy).
8. Antimetabolites: 6-mercaptopurine (an antimetabolite of adenine, it interferes with nucleic acid synthesis).

The enzymes which are inhibited by these drugs could obviously be used in systems to assay the drugs but, as far as I know, only cholinesterase has been used in this manner. Methods using cholinesterase for organophosphorous, halogenated, and carbamate pesticides as well as drugs have been published. Lipases (Guilbault and Sadar, 1969b) and acid and alkaline phosphatases (Guilbault *et al.*, 1969) have also been used for the estimation of pesticides.

Table 3. Enzymatic methods of drug analysis using the drug as an inhibitor

Drug	*Tissue*	*Enzyme*	*Reference*
Digitoxin	Plasma	Adenosine triphosphatase	Burnett and Conklin (1968)
Digoxin	Plasma	Adenosine triphosphatase	Burnett and Conklin (1971)
Monoamine oxidase inhibitors	Plasma and urine	Rat liver mitochondrial monoamine oxidase	Curry and Mercier (1970) Mercier and Curry (1971)
Heparin	Plasma	Ribonuclease	Zöllner and Lorenz (1965)
	Plasma	Pyruvate kinase	Horn (1965)
Ascorbic acid		Catalase	Orr (1966)

Table 3 lists drug assays involving inhibition methods, most of which can detect down to 10 ng. of the drug. The fact that both digoxin and digitoxin can be assayed by inhibiting the action of ATPase indicates the non-specificity of methods of this type. Obviously there will be a large range of organic compounds or even metal ions that will inhibit any given enzyme system. One corollary to this is that more than one enzyme system can be used to detect the drug; as, for example, in the case of heparin (*Table* 3).

The method of detecting monoamine oxidase inhibitors (Curry and Mercier, 1970; Mercier and Curry, 1971) solves this non-specificity by combining a thin-layer chromatographic separation with the inhibition of the enzyme. After extracting the drug from plasma or urine, the organic solvent is evaporated and spotted on to a

Silica Gel G thin-layer plate and developed using an ethyl acetate : chloroform mixture (1:1). The plate is then sprayed with a solution of monoamine oxidase (from rat liver mitochondria), and incubated for 15 minutes at 37° C. in a moisture tank to ensure satisfactory inhibition of the enzyme. To detect the spots due to the monoamine oxidase inhibitors, the plate is sprayed with a solution containing a tetrazolium salt and tryptamine and then reincubated for 2 hours at 37°C. The monoamine oxidase converts the tryptamine to the corresponding aldehyde which reacts with the colourless tetrazolium salt to form a blue formazan. The areas of inhibition therefore show as white spots on a blue background. The method can detect 10 ng. of these drugs.

Unlike those assays mentioned previously using the drug as a substrate (when either total change or kinetic methods could be used), when using the drug as an inhibitor only kinetic methods are applicable. The rate of the reaction is measured

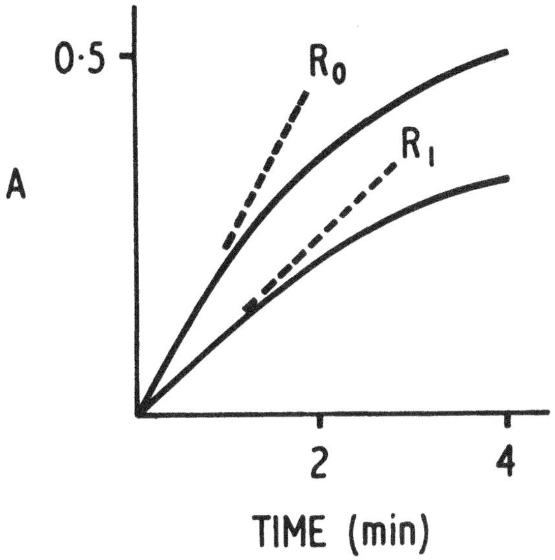

Fig. 4. The progress of a dehydrogenase reaction. R_0, rate of uninhibited system; R_I, rate of inhibited system.

as usual (e.g. in a dehydrogenase system using NAD, Δ absorbance/unit time would be measured) and then with the inhibitor added (*Fig.* 4). The percentage inhibition is then calculated from the equation:

$$\text{Percentage inhibition} = \frac{100\left(\begin{matrix}\text{Rate of the}\\ \text{uninhibited reaction}\end{matrix} - \begin{matrix}\text{Rate of the}\\ \text{inhibition reaction}\end{matrix}\right)}{\text{Rate of the uninhibited reaction}}$$

A calibration curve of percentage inhibition against concentration of inhibitor can then be constructed. For detection purposes it is only necessary to detect some inhibition of the system, but since this inhibition is usually not specific to a single substance, unless the drug can be identified by some other means, a number of enzyme systems must be used for the identification.

One system being developed at Birmingham University for the Home Office will use such a variety of systems (Townshend and O'Neill, 1972). To date only two systems have been examined in detail (*Table* 4), the limits of detection for the drugs

Table 4. The inhibition of enzyme systems by drugs (Townshend and O'Neill, 1972)

Drug	*Inhibition of enzyme at* $\leqslant 1 \times 10^{-6}$ g. per ml. Alcohol dehydrogenase	Lactate dehydrogenase
Lysergic acid diethylamide	+	+
Δ^9-Tetrahydrocannabinol	+	+
Morphine	+	–
Diamorphine	–	–
Phenobarbitone	–	–
Chlorpromazine	ND	+
Ascorbic acid	ND	+

\+ = Inhibition
– = No detectable inhibition
ND = Not done

being about 1 μg. per ml. In the case of the lactate dehydrogenase system, the forward and reverse reactions are both inhibited to the same extent. If many such enzyme systems could be used then this may be a way to identify a drug. A sample of blood or urine would be boiled to remove enzyme activity and an aliquot placed in a number of reaction tubes each containing a different enzyme. From those tubes showing inhibition a tentative identity could be assigned to the drug.

In many of the methods mentioned above, either when the drug is the substrate or when acting as an inhibitor, the end product is NADH and it is this that is measured. Thus, increasing the sensitivity of detection of NADH also increases the sensitivity of detection of the drug.

NADH Measurement

1. Using a direct ultra-violet (UV) measurement at 340 nm., NADH has a molar extinction coefficient of $6{\cdot}22 \times 10^3$; i.e. in a 1-cm. cell a solution containing 1 μg. per ml. has an absorbance of about 0·001.

2. Coupled reactions can be used, e.g.

$$\text{NADH} + \underset{\text{(Colourless)}}{\underset{\text{violet}}{p\text{-Iodonitrotetrazolium}}} \xrightarrow[\quad]{\substack{\text{Phenazine}\\ \text{methosulphate}}} \underset{\text{(Coloured)}}{\text{Formazan}}$$

In this case the colourless tetrazolium salt is converted by NADH to the coloured formazan (which can be read at 520 nm.) (Whitaker, 1969). Phenazine methosulphate (PMS) is used as an electron transfer agent. The sensitivity of detection is not markedly increased, but since the reaction is visible the advantages are that a simple colorimeter can be used instead of a UV spectrophotometer and the reagent can be used as a TLC spray (as for the monoamine oxidase inhibitors). Formazan formation has also been used for the assay of ethanol in blood (Léric *et al.*, 1970).

3. Fluorometric methods give greater sensitivity without much increase in practical difficulty. The direct measurement by exciting at 340 nm. and measuring the emission at 450 nm. gives a x10 increase in sensitivity over the UV method. If the measurement is made in 6*N* sodium hydroxide solution, a further increase in sensitivity is obtained (Townshend and O'Neill, 1972).

4. Indirect fluorescent methods can be used by means of coupled reactions. The non-fluorescent compound resazurin can be converted to the fluorescent compound

resorufin by NADH easily and quantitatively using either PMS or diaphorase (*Fig.* 5). The excitation wavelength is 560 nm., the emission is measured at 580 nm.,

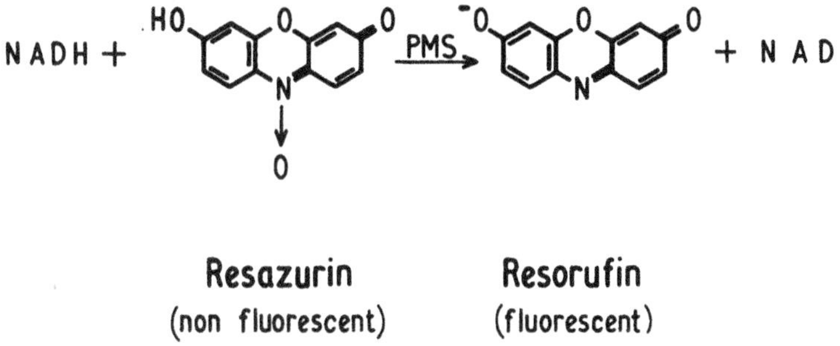

Fig. 5. Coupled reaction for the indirect fluorometric measurement of NADH.

and the calibration is ΔF. per min. versus concentration of NADH. By this means from 2×10^{-7} to 2×10^{-5} *M* NADH can be measured with a standard deviation of 0·5 per cent (Guilbault and Kramer, 1965). The method is claimed to have an increase in sensitivity over direct fluorometric measurement of between 10 and 100.

5. The above fluorometric methods can detect down to 10^{-11} moles per ml. NADH. Increased sensitivity by several orders may be obtained by using an enzyme cycling technique (Lowry *et al.,* 1961). *Fig.* 6 illustrates one such system. If we

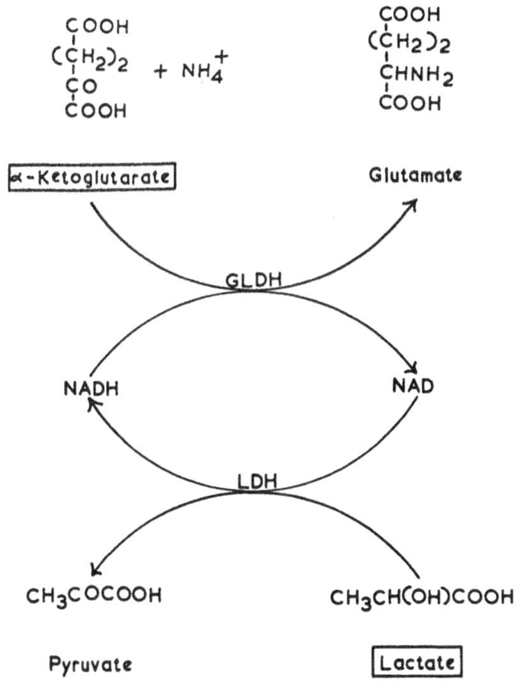

Fig. 6. Enzyme cycling reaction for the measurement of NADH (GLDH, glutamate dehydrogenase; LDH, lactate dehydrogenase).

assume that NADH has already been produced by one of the reactions mentioned earlier it is necessary to treat the incubation medium with mild alkali in order to destroy the enzyme that was used and any unconverted NAD. (Conversely if NAD is being assayed, brief acid treatment would destroy any remaining NADH and enzyme activity.) To the solution containing the NADH is added α-ketoglutarate, glutamate dehydrogenase (GLDH), lactate dehydrogenase (LDH), and lactate. The solution is then incubated at 25°C. for 30 minutes. The α-ketoglutarate is converted by the GLDH and NADH to glutamate with the production of NAD. This is subsequently reconverted to NADH by LDH with the associated conversion of lactate to pyruvate. The reaction is stopped by heating in a boiling water bath. The amount of pyruvate produced is measured in a second step with added NADH and LDH.

If the nucleotides are used at concentrations well below their Michaelis Constants the final concentration of pyruvate is directly proportional to the original concentration of NADH. It is in from 10^3 to 10^4 greater quantity than the original NADH and therefore increases the sensitivity of detection by this amount. Since the final product is also a nucleotide, the cyclic process could be repeated again and again.

So far this paper has been concerned with the use of enzymes in *in vitro* detection systems. Since the drugs have an obvious effect on the body it is conceivable that their detection and identification can also be achieved by studying the results of their actions *in vivo.*

BIOCHEMICAL LESIONS

In every cell in the body the activities of the enzymes and the concentrations of the substrates to which they pertain are maintained at relatively constant levels by a balance of synthesis and degradation. When drugs alter this balance to cause the death of the organism they often do it by altering the levels of these enzymes. The biochemical lesions caused by such drugs might therefore be demonstrated if the enzymes concerned are long lived or if their activities before death could be estimated from the levels of the substrates on which they act or on the products of the enzymatic reaction.

Drugs affecting enzymes can act in many different ways when given in therapeutic doses:

1. Increase the amount or activity of an enzyme present in an organ by inducing metabolism; e.g. phenobarbitone with microsomal enzymes.
2. Reduce enzyme efficiency by competitive inhibition.
3. Permanently reduce the efficiency; e.g. monoamine oxidase inhibitors where the effect does not reach a maximum until two weeks after commencement of treatment.

However, in acute poisoning the drug affecting the enzyme nearly always acts as an inhibitor. We are looking at several systems to see firstly if a range of normal values can be obtained for various different systems and then to see if acute poisoning changes these values in a recognizable and reproducible manner.

From the distribution of results that we get (*Fig.* 7) we will have to sort the 'normals' from those in hypo- or hyper-active conditions due to a disease state; e.g. an inborn error of metabolism or temporary infection, etc. Hopefully we will then be able to distinguish these three conditions from the extremes which would correspond to activities pushed to their limits by acute overdosage of drugs.

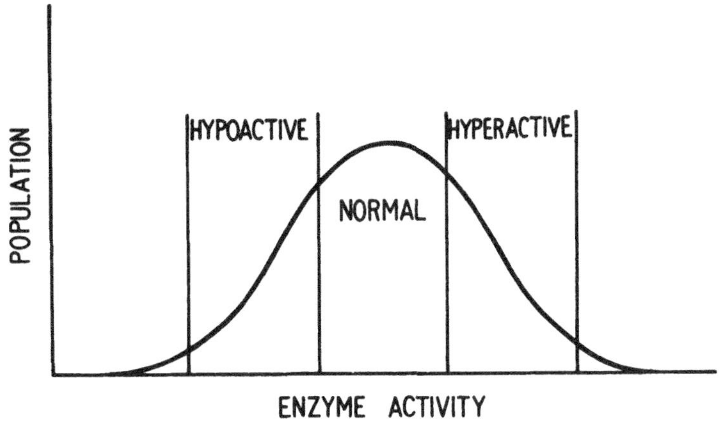

Fig. 7. Hypothetical distribution of the activity of an enzyme within individuals of a population.

That is our philosophy and the systems on which we are working are discussed below. *Fig.* 8 illustrates the well known primary pathways of metabolism of the

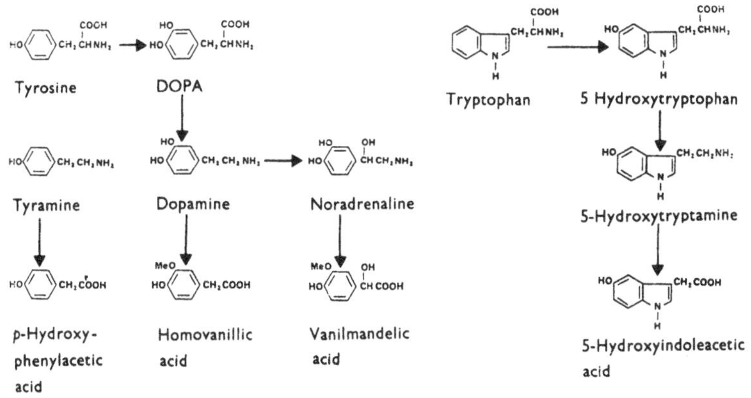

Fig. 8. Primary metabolic pathways of some brain amines.

brain amines. The amino-acids tyrosine and tryptophan are both hydroxylated and then decarboxylated to give dopamine and 5-hydroxytryptamine respectively. Dopamine is further converted to noradrenaline. Tyramine, dopamine, noradrenaline and 5-hydroxytryptamine are then all converted by monoamine oxidase, catechol-*O*-methyl transferase and aldehyde oxidase to their respective carboxylic acids; *viz, p*-hydroxyphenylacetic acid (*p*HPAA), homovanillic acid (HVA), vanilmandelic acid (VMA) and 5-hydroxyindoleacetic acid (5-HIAA). The concentrations of these acids may be used to monitor the turnover of the brain amines and thus the activities of the enzymes. (Turnover here would include release mechanisms as well as the usual metabolism.) Blockade of the anabolic routes of the amines would obviously decrease the concentration of amines in the brain, whereas the reverse would be true if the catabolic pathways were blocked or reduced in efficiency. (Although this paper is concerned with enzymes, this type of approach would obviously include all drugs which affect brain amines whether they act by means of altering enzyme levels or by changing the release, leakage, or uptake of the amines from the cell.)

Monoamine oxidase inhibitors are the drugs in which we are most interested, partly because they are difficult to detect chemically and partly because sufficient work has already been carried out to ensure that this project is a viable proposition. Apart from examining the level of monoamine oxidase in the hind brain, the levels of the substrates can be used to detect changes in enzyme activities. For example, in patients who died from non-drug causes the post-mortem brain levels of 5-hydroxytryptamine, noradrenaline, and dopamine were raised by factors of two or three in patients receiving monoamine oxidase inhibitors for depression compared with controls (*Table* 5). It is reasonable to assume that acute poisonings involving monoamine oxidase inhibitors would show even greater differences from controls.

Table 5. Post-mortem brain levels of monoamines in patients receiving therapeutic doses of monoamine oxidase inhibitors and controls all of whom died from non-drug causes.*

Drug	*Mean concentration of monoamines in brain* (μg. per g.)		
	5-Hydroxytryptamine (brain-stem)	Noradrenaline (hypothalamus)	Dopamine (hypothalamus)
Isocarboxazid	0·80	0·93	0·36
Pargyline	0·84	1·53	0·36
Tranylcypromine	1·00	1·46	0·56
Controls	0·39	0·49	0·25

* From Bevan-Jones *et al.* Reproduced by permission of the Editor, *British Medical Journal.*

We thought that the concentration of the acid metabolites of the amines in the urine would be a good measure of the turnover of the parent amines in the brain, so we collected a large number of urine samples from different individuals and analysed them by gas chromatography. The samples were extracted, evaporated to dryness, derivatized and chromatographed on a DC 560 column programmed from 100 to 220°C. at 2° per minute. A good separation was obtained and the peaks were identified from standards run previously (*Fig.* 9). Identities can be assigned to all

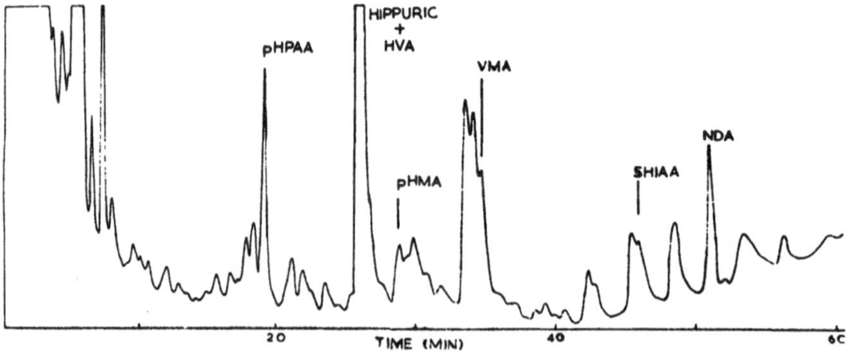

Fig. 9. Chromatogram of the methyl esters – trimethylsilyl ethers of an acid extract of human urine on a 5 per cent DC 560 column programmed from 100 to 220°C. at 2°C. per min. (pHPAA, para-hydroxyphenylacetic acid; HVA, homovanillic acid; pHMA, para-hydroxymandelic acid; VMA, vanilmandelic acid; 5HIAA, 5-hydroxyindoleacetic acid; NDA, nonadecanoic acid, internal standard).

the peaks on the basis of the retention times (or more correctly methylene units) from the work of Dalgliesh *et al.* (1966). The first results we obtained were very encouraging (*Fig.* 10) and there were very few differences in the chromatograms.

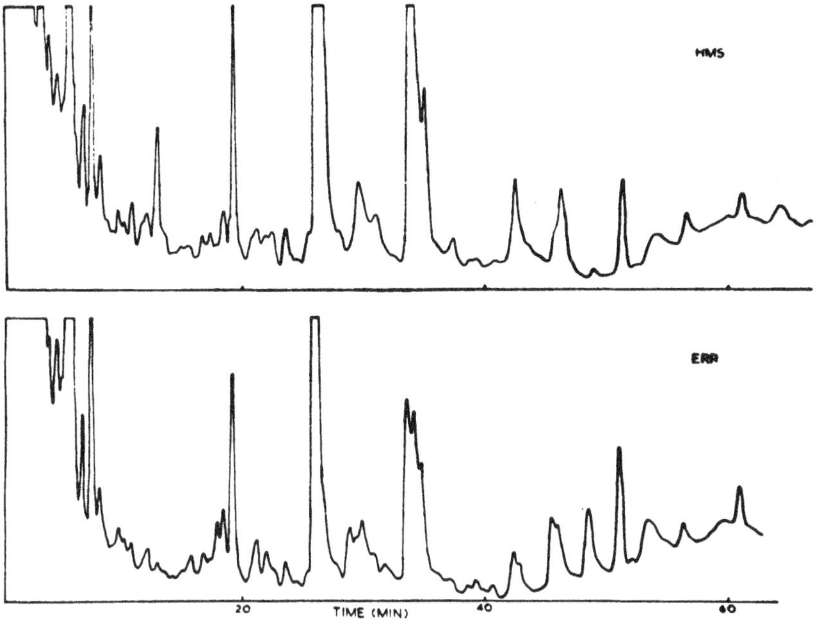

Fig. 10. Chromatograms of the methyl esters – trimethylsilyl ethers of the acid extracts of urine from subjects HMS and ERR.

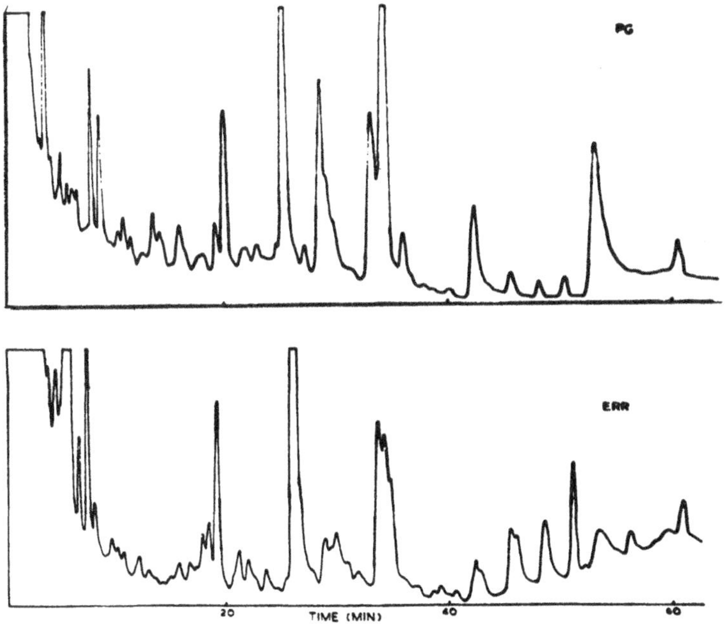

Fig. 11. Chromatograms of the methyl esters – trimethylsilyl ethers of the acid extracts of urines from subjects PG and ERR.

However, as we obtained more samples, some of the later chromatograms were not comparable to those obtained previously (*Fig.* 11). Analysing samples obtained from the same individual on different occasions also gave far from a constant picture (*Fig.* 12). We are therefore changing to measuring brain levels of these compounds and are in the midst of working up the methodology for estimating the brain amines, acid metabolites, and monoamine oxidase at the moment.

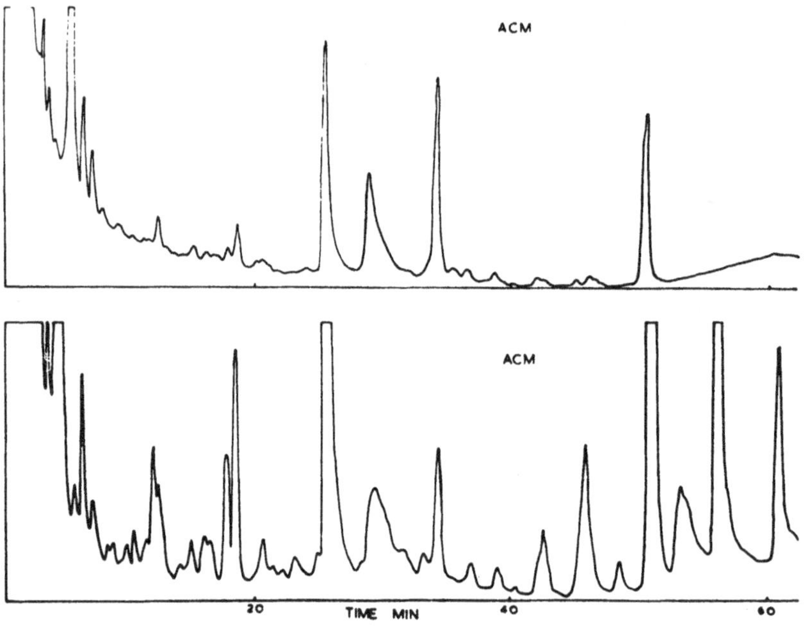

Fig. 12. Chromatograms of the methyl esters – trimethylsilyl ethers of the acid extracts of urine from one subject obtained on consecutive days.

3′, 5′-Cyclic adenosine monophosphate (cAMP) is the popular biochemical for research these days and the excretion in the urine has been shown to reflect the state of mind (Abdulla and Hamadah, 1970). Thus, the urinary levels of cAMP should reflect any brain disturbance, and this is another of the systems at which we are looking. An extracellular hormone (*see Fig.* 13) attaches itself to the receptor so activating the adenyl cyclase attached to the cell membrane. This enzyme catalyses the intracellular conversion of adenosine triphosphate (ATP) to cAMP, and it is the cAMP which causes the response within the cell; i.e. it acts as a second messenger. The enzyme responsible for the destruction of cAMP to the inactive 5′-adenosine monophosphate (5′-AMP) is phosphodiesterase. We have examined the effects of 70 drugs on an *in vitro* system containing phosphodiesterase and found that amongst the most potent inhibitors are some of the antidepressent drugs, *viz* trifluoperazine and triflupromazine (Moffat *et al.,* 1972). It may well be that these antidepressants exert part of their action by this means.

An isotope dilution method of assay using a specific binding protein is being used to assay the cAMP in urine and we are at the moment collecting urine samples from patients whose cause of death was acute overdosage of known drugs. At the same time we are also collecting and analysing samples from people who died from natural causes, and will later compare the two sets of data and correlate them with the research on the phosphodiesterase inhibitors.

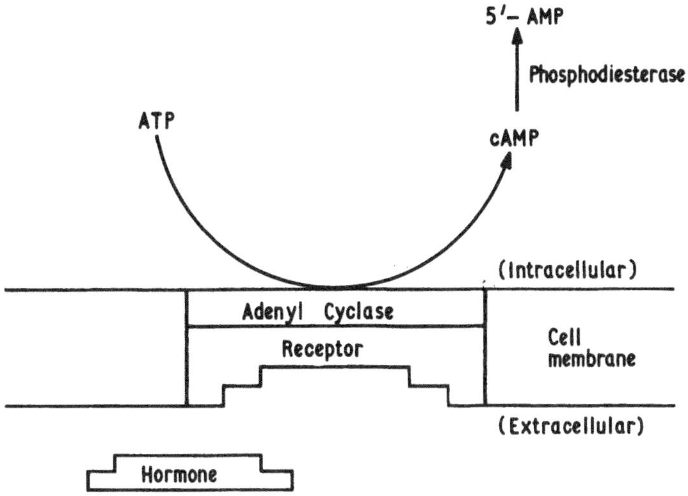

Fig. 13. Diagram of the synthesis and destruction of cAMP within a cell. (ATP, adenosine triphosphate; cAMP, 3′, 5′-cyclic adenosine monophosphate; 5′-AMP, 5′-adenosine monophosphate.)

Serum levels of cholinesterase can be used to monitor the toxic effects of anti-cholinesterases. Refrigerated samples are stable for several weeks so the enzyme levels can be determined many days after death has occurred. One method used as routine in forensic science laboratories is as follows:

Buffer solution (2·5 ml., *p*H 8·0) and substrate solution (2·5 ml. of an aqueous solution containing 50 mg. of acetylcholine bromide) are placed in two tubes and 50 μl. serum or whole blood is added to one tube. The *p*H of each solution is read immediately and again after incubation at 25°C. for one hour. The difference in *p*H between the control and the incubated blood x100 gives the cholinesterase activity in *p*H units (Michel, 1949). Normal whole blood gives values of 80–160 *p*H units.

Other serum enzyme levels are used to obtain information valuable for diagnosis and for following the course of many diseases. The enzymes most commonly examined are given in *Table* 6. Increases in serum enzyme activities above the normal range occur when cells are damaged by disease or drugs and their membranes leak enzymes into the blood. Enzyme levels are then proportional to the tissue damage. The organs most affected are the liver, heart, and pancreas. Studies on experimental animals have shown that there is a far reaching correlation between the increase in

Table 6. Serum enzymes whose activities in serum are valuable in diagnosis

Acid phosphatase (SP)
Alkaline phosphatase (AP)
α-Amylase (diastase);
Aldolase (ALD)
Creatine phosphokinase (CPK)
Glutamate dehydrogenase (GLDH)
Glutamate-oxaloacetate transaminase (GOT)
Glutamate-pyruvate transaminase (GPT)
Lactate dehydrogenase (LDH)

activity of individual enzymes (particularly transaminases) and the dose of a toxin (Schmidt *et al.*, 1965). Also, after hypoxia there is a considerable rise in the serum enzyme activities after a short time, although the structural changes are only visible after 4–6 hours. Serum creatine phosphokinase is also elevated in patients after overdosage of hypnotic or tricyclic antidepressant drugs (Wright *et al.*, 1971).

After death, autolysis would change the blood picture drastically so that post-mortem serum enzyme levels would probably not be useful in diagnosing different types of poisoning. However, the enzyme activity of urine may not be affected too much and we are just starting a short research project to see if post-mortem urinary enzyme levels can be linked to particular types of poisoning. Some research in this field has already been carried out, although most of the drugs examined were nephrotoxic. For example, alkaline phosphatase activity in urine increases after the administration of aspirin or aspirin and caffeine to rats (*Fig.* 14).

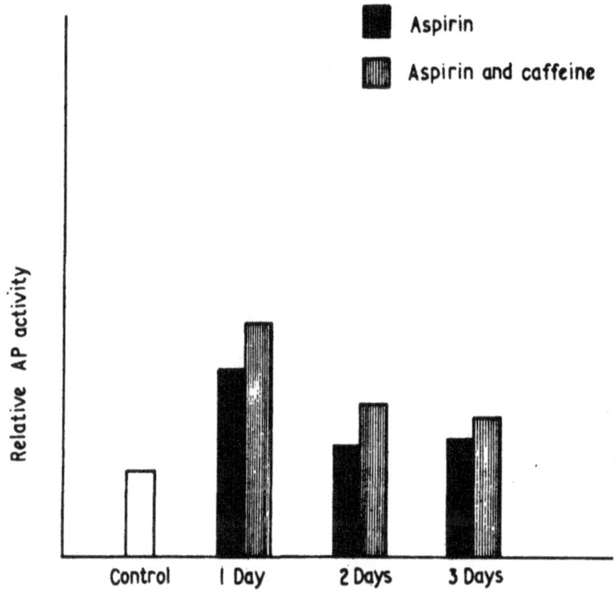

Fig. 14 Alkaline phosphatase (AP) activity in the supernatant urine of rats before and after the oral administration of aspirin (100 mg. per kg.) or aspirin (100 mg. per kg.) and caffeine (50 mg. per kg.). (From Raab, 1972; rep duced by permission of *Clinical Chemistry.*)

Other urinary enzyme levels have also been reported to be raised after drug toxicity; lactate dehydrogenase by streptomycin, kanamycin, and aspirin (Plummer and Leathwood, 1968; Leathwood and Plummer, 1969; Raab, 1970) and leucine aminopeptidase by sulphonamides (Raab and Hohenegger, 1968).

The presence of enzymes in urine is not always a help. In our studies with succinylcholine we noticed that standard solutions made up in samples of my urine contained no detectable succinylcholine after they had been left on the bench for a few minutes (Stevens, H. M. and Moffat, A. C., unpublished observations). However, if the urine was first boiled to remove any cholinesterase activity before the solution was made, the drug could then be detected.

In spite of the nuisance value of some enzymes as related above, I hope it has been shown that enzymes are useful reagents and can be used to detect drugs in many different ways. It is to be expected that in the future enzymatic tests for drugs will become even simpler and quicker and, because of their inherent specificity, become of even greater value to the practising forensic toxicologist.

REFERENCES

ABDULLA, Y. H., and HAMADAH, K. (1970), 3′, 5′-Cyclic adenosine monophosphate in depression and mania, *Lancet,* **1**, 378–381.

AMMON, R., and KAMPHUES, V. (1969), Anreicherung von dolantinesterase aus kaninchenleber, *Enzymologica,* **37**, 345–355.

BELL, G. H., DAVIDSON, J. N., and SCARBOROUGH, H. (1961), *Textbook of Physiology and Biochemistry,* 5th ed., p. 79. London: Livingstone.

BEVAN JONES, A. B., PARE, C. M. B., NICHOLSON, W. J., PRICE, K., and STACEY, R. S. (1972), Brain amine concentrations after monoamine oxidase inhibitor administration, *Br. med. J.,* **1**, 17–19.

BONNICHSEN, R. (1965), Ethanol – Determination with alcohol dehydrogenase and DPN. In *Methods of Enzymatic Analysis* (ed. BERGMEYER, H. V.), pp. 285–289. New York: Academic Press.

BRITISH PHARMACOPOEIA (1968), London: General Medical Council.

BURNETT, G. H., and CONKLIN, R. L. (1968), The enzymatic assay of plasma digitoxin levels, *J. Lab. clin. Med.,* **71**, 1040–1044.

—, — (1971), The enzymatic assay of plasma digoxin, *Ibid.,* **78**, 779–784.

CRAWHALL, J. C., and WATTS, R. W. E. (1961), The oxalate content of human plasma, *Clin. Sci.,* **20**, 357–366.

CURRY, A. S., and MERCIER, M. (1970), Detection and identification of monoamine oxidase inhibitors in biological samples, *Nature, Lond.,* **228**, 281.

DALGLIESH, C. E., HORNING, E. C., HORNING, M. G., KNOX, K. L., and YARGER, K. (1966), A gas-liquid chromatographic procedure for separating a wide range of metabolites occurring in urine or tissue extract, *Biochem. J.,* **101**, 792–810.

EXTRA PHARMACOPOEIA (1967), *Martindale* (ed. TODD, R. G.) 25th ed. London: Pharmaceutical Press.

GOLDBERG, L., and RYDBERG, U. (1965), Automated enzymatic micro-determination of ethanol in blood and urine. In *Automation in Analytical Chemistry* (ed. SKEGGS, L. T.), pp. 595–600. New York: Mediad.

GUILBAULT, G. G. (1968), Use of enzymes in analytical chemistry, *Analyt. Chem.,* **40**, 459R–471R.

—(1970), Use of enzymes in and kinetic aspects of analytical chemistry, *Ibid.,* **42**, 334R–349R.

—, and KRAMER, D. N. (1965), Fluorometric procedure for measuring the activity of dehydrogenases. *Ibid.,* **37**, 1219–1221.

—, and SADAR, S. H. (1969a), Fluorometric assay of alcohols using alcohol oxidase, *Analyt. Lett.,* **2**, 41–48.

—, — (1969b), Fluorometric determination of pesticides, *Analyt. Chem.,* **41**, 366–368.

—, —, and ZIMMER, M. (1969), Analytical applications of the phosphatase enzyme system – Determination of bismuth, beryllium and pesticides, *Analytica chim. Acta.,* **44**, 361–367.

HORN, H. D. (1965), Heparin – Determination with pyruvic kinase. In *Methods of Enzymatic Analysis* (ed. BERGMEYER, H. V.), pp. 84–86, New York: Academic Press.

HUBENER, H. J. (1965), Determination of 20-ketosteroids by a spectrophotometric method. In *Methods of Enzymatic Analysis* (ed. BERGMEYER, H. V.), pp. 477–480. New York: Academic Press.

JONES, D., GERBER, L. P., and DRELL, W. (1970), A rapid enzymatic method for estimating ethanol in body fluids, *Clin. Chem.*, **16**, 402–407.

LEATHWOOD, P. D., and PLUMMER, D. T. (1969), The excretion of lactate dehydrogenase in human urine after the ingestion of aspirin, *Biochem, J.*, **114**, 197–202.

LERIC, H., KAPLAN, J. C., and BROUN, G. (1970), Dosage enzymatique de l'alcool sanguin par microméthode colorimétrique, *Clin. Chim. Acta*, **29**, 523–528.

LOWRY, O. H., PASSONNEAU, J. V., SCHULZ, D. W., and ROCK, M. K. (1961), The measurement of pyridine nucleotides by enzymatic cycling, *J. biol. Chem.*, **236**, 2746–2755.

MARUYAMA, H., and COURSIN, D. B. (1968), Enzymic assay of pyridoxal phosphate using tyrosine apodecarboxylase and tyrosine-1-^{14}C, *Analyt. Biochem.*, **26**, 420–429.

MAYER, G. G., MARKOW, D., and KARP, F. (1963), Enzymatic oxalate determination in urine, *Clin. Chem.*, **9**, 334–339.

MERCIER, M. J., and CURRY, A. S. (1971), Méthode enzymatique pour la recherche des inhibiteurs de la monoamine oxydase, *European J. Tox.*, **4**, 36–38.

MICHEL, H. O. (1949), An electrometric method for the determination of red blood cell and plasma cholinesterase activity, *J. Lab. clin. Med.*, **34**, 1564–1568.

MOFFAT, A. C., PATTERSON, D. A., CURRY, A. S., and OWEN, P. (1972), Inhibition in vitro of cyclic 3′,5′-nucleotide phosphodiesterase activity by drugs, *European J. Tox.*, **5**, 160–162.

ORR, C. W. M. (1966), The inhibition of catalase by ascorbic acid, *Biochem. biophys. Res Commun.*, **23**, 854–860.

PLUMMER, D. T., and LEATHWOOD, P. D. (1968), The effect of salicylate on urinary lactate dehydrogenase, *Biochem. J.*, **106**, 55P–56P.

RAAB, W. P. (1970), Renal effects of streptomycin in rats, *Clinica. chim. Acta*, **29**, 451–454.

— (1972), Diagnostic value of urinary enzyme determinations, *Clin. Chem.*, **18**, 5–25.

—, and HOHENEGGER, M. (1968), Renale enzymausscheidung bei ratten nach hohen dosen von penicillin, kanamycin und sulphonamiden, *Clinica. chim. Acta*, **20**, 95–103.

RIBEIRO, M. E., and ELLIOT, J. S. (1964), Direct enzymatic determination of urinary oxalate, *Invest. Urol.*, **2**, 78–81.

SCHMIDT, E., SCHMIDT, F. W., HORN, H. D., and GERLACH, U. (1965), The importance of the measurement of enzyme activity in medicine. In *Methods of Enzymatic Analysis* (ed. BERGMEYER, H. V.), p. 651–665. New York: Academic Press.

SEILER, V. N., and WERNER, G. (1965), An enzymatic method for the determination of the racemisation rate of hyoscyamine and scopolamine, *Arzneimittel-Forsch.*, **15**, 189.

THURSTON, J. H., LIANG, H. S., SMITH, J. S., and VALENTINI, E. J. (1968), New enzymatic method for measurement of paraldehyde: Correlation of effects with serum and CSF levels, *J. Lab. clin. Med.*, 72, 699–704.

TOWNSHEND, A., and O'NEILL, R. B. (1972), Personal communication.

WADE, H. E. (1972), Personal communication.

WHITAKER, J. F. (1969), A general colorimetric procedure for the estimation of enzymes which are linked to the NADH/NAD^+ system. *Clinica. chim. Acta,* **24**, 23–37.

WRIGHT, N., CLARKSON, A. R., BROWN, S. S., and FUSTER, V. (1971), Effects of poisoning on serum enzyme activities, coagulation and fibrinolysis, *Br. med. J.*, **3**, 347–350.

ZÖLLNER, N., and LORENZ, B. (1965), Heparin – Determination with ribonuclease. In *Methods of Enzymatic Analysis* (ed. BERGMEYER, H. V.), pp. 79–82. New York: Academic Press.

Rapid Tests for Drugs in Urine

E. G. C. CLARKE
Department of Physiology, The Royal Veterinary College, London

Most chemical analyses arising from drug addiction call for a rapid answer, but a toxicological laboratory handling a heavy work-load is usually unable to supply this. Accordingly, during the last few years there have been introduced a number of so-called simple methods for the detection of drugs (Baden *et al.*, 1972; Bastos *et al.*, 1970; Beckett *et al.*, 1967; Berry *et al.*, 1970; Bowen *et al.*, 1970; Broich *et al.*, 1971; Davidow *et al.*, 1968; Dole *et al.*, 1966, 1972; Garriott and Stolman, 1971; Ho *et al.*, 1972; Marks *et al.*, 1969; Mulé, 1969; Ono *et al.*, 1969; Ramsey and

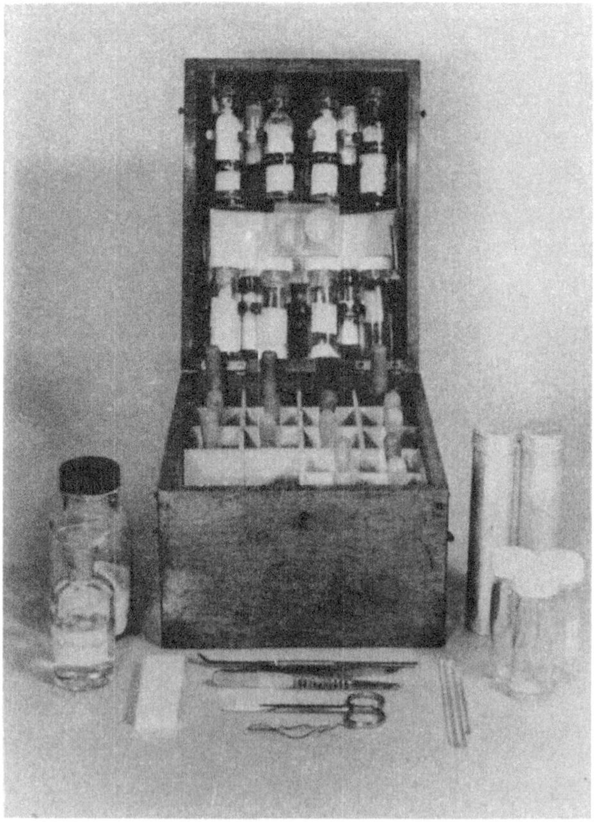

Fig. 1. Equipment and reagent bottles used in the rapid tests for drugs in urine. The equipment and reagents required are listed in *Table* 1.

Campbell, 1971; Steel *et al.*, 1970). Even these methods, however, presuppose the availability of a well-trained chemist with reasonable laboratory facilities, and even the simplest technique described might well take several hours to perform. There are, however, occasions when neither time nor facilities are available. For example, the physician at an addiction treatment centre may want to know if the patient he is interviewing is keeping to the prescribed methadone, or whether he has relapsed to clandestine heroin. A urine test is indicated, but a laboratory is unlikely to be able to furnish the result of this in less than 24 hours. What is needed is an immediate answer, available while the interview is still in progress. This seems to indicate the need for some test that can be carried out on the spot by a nurse or a receptionist with no special training and the minimum of equipment. The method described below was evolved in an attempt to fill this need. It is in no way intended as a substitute for existing forms of analysis, nor to stand up to cross-examination in a court of law. It is primarily intended for urine, but may be used for tablets, capsules etc. by crushing them, mixing with water and a little dilute sulphuric acid, and treating the resulting solution or suspension as though it were urine.

The equipment needed for carrying out the tests can be contained in a box 25 x 20 x 20 cm., and weighing less than 4 kg. (*Fig.* 1). The contents of the box are given in *Table* 1.

Table 1. Equipment and reagents required for the rapid detection of drugs in urine.

Equipment:
One 6-oz. wide-mouthed screw capped bottle
Several McCartney bottles
Several small white tiles
Glass rods
A small porcelain basin
20 gauge copper wire
Strips of No. 1 Whatman filter paper, 1 cm. wide
Forceps
Scissors

Solid compounds:
Anhydrous sodium sulphate
Sodium tetraborate
Sulphamic acid
N-1-naphthyl ethylene diamine dihydrochloride

Dropping bottles containing reagents:
Concentrated sulphuric acid
Concentrated hydrochloric acid[1]
2 *N* sulphuric acid
Marquis reagent (2 per cent paraformaldehyde in concentrated sulphuric acid)
Potassium iodoplatinate solution (2·5 per cent)
Sodium sulphite solution (10 per cent, freshly prepared)
FPN reagent
Cobalt thiocyanate solution (2 per cent)
Ammonium vanadate solution (saturated, in 5 *N* ammonium hydroxide solution)
Sodium nitrite solution (0·1 per cent, freshly prepared)
Sulphuric acid solution (0·5 per cent)[2]
N-1-naphthylethylene diamine dihydrochloride solution (0·1 per cent)
Acetone/water (20:1, for chromatography)[1]

[1] These should be in bottles with pipettes graduated at 1 ml.
[2] In a bottle with a pipette drawn out to a fine point.

Basic drugs are extracted as follows (Clarke, 1971). The McCartney bottle serves as a measure. Pour this volume of chloroform into a 6-oz. bottle containing 75 g. of anhydrous sodium sulphate and 1 g. of borax. Shake briefly and then add an equal volume of urine. Shake thoroughly and pour the chloroform off into a McCartney bottle. Re-extract the urine/sulphate mixture with half the above volume of chloroform and add this to the original extract. Dry by shaking with a little anhydrous sodium sulphate, and decant into another McCartney bottle. Basic compounds are now extracted from the chloroform by the acid-spot method (Morgan, 1959). Take a strip of filter paper 15 x 1 cm. and spot it with dilute sulphuric acid at 2 cm. intervals, the end spots being 2·5 cm. from the ends of the strip (*Fig.* 2). Fold the paper and immerse it in the chloroform. It must now be

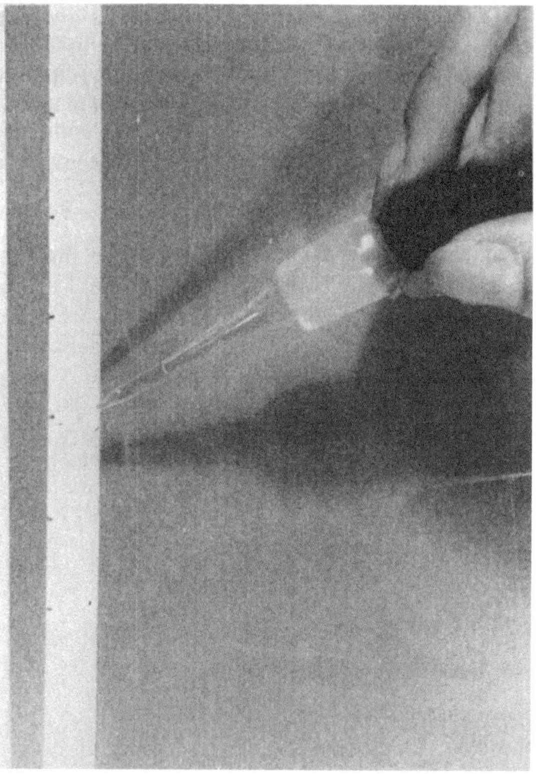

Fig. 2. Method of spotting filter paper with dilute sulphuric acid in the acid-spot method for extracting basic compounds from chloroform. The interval between the spots is 2 cm., and the end spots are 2·5 cm. from the ends of the strip.

shaken for at least ten minutes, preferably longer; alternatively, it can be allowed to stand overnight.

Remove the paper, allow it to dry, and cut it up. The two longer end pieces are kept for subsequent chromatography, while the four short pieces are used for colour tests. A colour with iodoplatinate indicates that some basic drug is present; it may be nicotine. Further information may be obtained by adding a drop of sodium sulphite solution to the iodoplatinate spot. Nicotine and morphine bleach almost immediately but methadone and certain other drugs, for example, amitriptylene and imipramine, turn reddish and fade very slowly, taking 15 minutes or more. The next spot is tested with the Marquis reagent. A purple colour is given by morphine and the phenothiazines, orange turning to brown by amphetamine, and yellow by the benzhydryl derivatives. If the third spot is treated with the concentrated sulphuric acid it will help to differentiate, as the phenothiazines and benzhydryl drugs such as diphenhydramine give the same colour as with the Marquis reagent, but morphine and amphetamine give no colour. Other tests, such as the FPN reagent, the cobalt thiocyanate test, and the ammonium vanadate/sulphuric acid test can be carried out on the remaining spots.

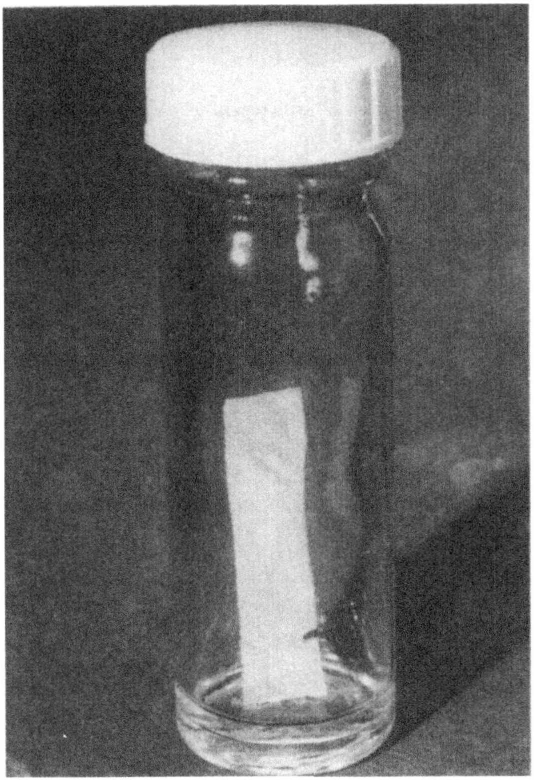

Fig. 3. Microscale paper chromotography in acetone/water (20:1) performed in McCartney bottles.

In the case of suspected mixtures, separation can be effected by running microscale paper chromatograms in acetone/water (20:1) in McCartney bottles, using the longer pieces of paper carrying the acid spots (*Fig.* 3). After about a minute, when the solvent front will have risen about 1·5 cm., the paper is removed, dried, and treated with the appropriate reagent. Nicotine and morphine, for example, remain on the baseline, while methadone runs at the solvent front.

Of the benzodiazepine drugs, only nitrazepam can be detected on an acid spot obtained as above. This is because it is metabolized, at any rate in part, to the 7-amino derivative (*Fig.* 4), which is a reasonably strong base (Pribilla, 1965;

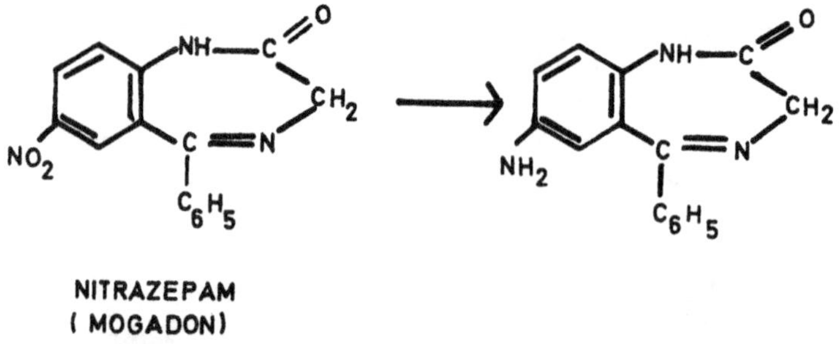

Fig. 4. Metabolism of nitrazepam to 7-aminonitrazepam.

Reider, 1965; Thompsett, 1968). It is extracted from chloroform by dilute acid, and gives a Bratton-Marshall test (Bratton and Marshall, 1939). This may be carried out in an ignition tube or a small porcelain basin. Add two drops of dilute sulphuric acid to the acid spot, then one drop of sodium nitrite solution, wait half a minute, then add a drop of sulphamic acid solution, wait another half minute, then finally add a drop of *N*-1-naphthyl ethylene diamine dihydrochloride solution, shaking or stirring after each addition. A magenta colour forms slowly.

The other benzodiazepines cannot be detected in this simple way as neither they nor their metabolites can be extracted by the acid-spot method. It is necessary to carry out hydrolysis first. Chlordiazepoxide (Koechlin and d'Arconte, 1963; Koechlin *et al.*, 1965) is metabolized in the body to the 'lactam' which on acid hydrolysis yields 2-amino-7-chloro-benzophenone (ACB) (*Fig.* 5). Note that the

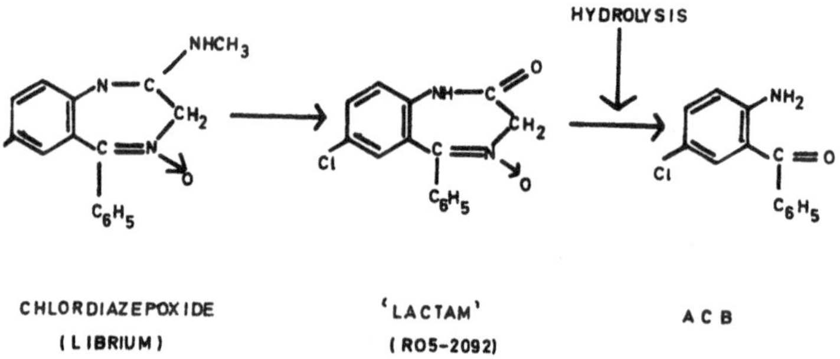

Fig. 5. Chlordiazepoxide is metabolized in the body to 'Lactam'. To allow extraction by the acid-spot method it is necessary to carry out hydrolysis first, resulting in the production of 2-amino-7-chloro-benzophenone (ACB).

metabolic pathways given here are only those relevant to the detection of these drugs in urine by the method being described. Diazepam (Schwartz *et al.*, 1965; de Silva *et al.*, 1966; de Silva and Puglizi, 1970) is demethylated and then hydroxylated to give oxazepam, which is present in urine as the glucuronide (*Fig.* 6).

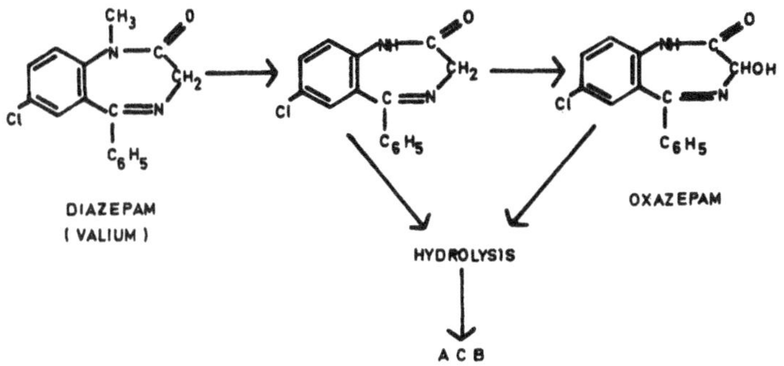

Fig. 6. Diazepam is metabolized by demethylation followed by hydroxylation to yield oxazepam, which is present in urine as the glucuronide. Acid hydrolysis splits the glucuronide and converts both demethylated diazepam and oxazepam to 2-amino-7-chloro-benzophenone (ACB).

This may be split by acid hydrolysis, which will further convert both oxazepam and demethylated diazepam to ACB (Walkenstein *et al.*, 1964; Weist, 1968; Pelzer and Maass, 1969). Medazepam (Schwartz and Carbone, 1970: de Silva and Puglizi, 1970) is metabolized to diazepam which then follows the same pathway (*Fig.* 7). Thus, the end product of all these compounds is ACB, which, having a primary arylamino group, gives a Bratton-Marshall reaction, and thus affords a means of detection. This is carried out as follows:

Take 4 ml. of urine in a McCartney bottle. Add 1 ml. of concentrated HCl. Heat on a boiling water bath for half an hour. Under field conditions, a saucepan or an

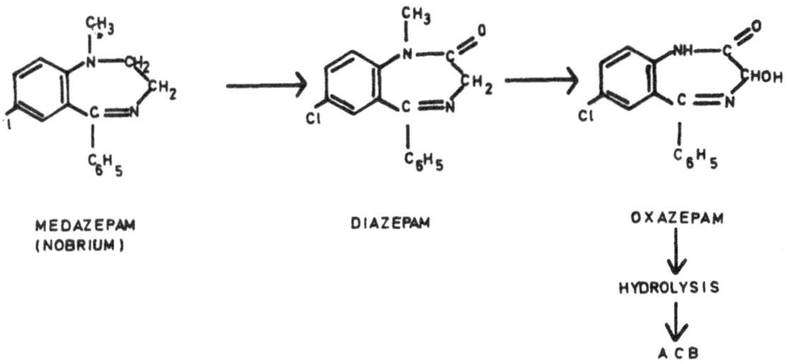

Fig. 7. Metabolism of medazepam to diazepam and thence to oxazepam, as shown in *Fig.* 6. Acid hydrolysis yields 2-amino-7-chloro-benzophenone (ACB).

electric kettle can be used, the bottle being kept upright by a copper wire twisted round its neck and bent over the side of the vessel. One can even carry out the hydrolysis by lowering the McCartney bottle into a vacuum flask, surrounding it with boiling water, and allowing it to stand. Remove the bottle, cool and make alkaline by adding 10 pellets of sodium hydroxide. Pour into a McCartney bottle half full of anhydrous sodium sulphate to which chloroform has been added until there is a layer 0·5 cm. deep on top of the sulphate. Shake, and decant the chloroform into a small porcelain dish. As ACB is very soluble in chloroform, and is only weakly basic, it cannot be extracted by an acid spot, so it is necessary to evaporate the solution and do the Bratton-Marshall test on the residue. Add two drops of dilute acid, stir with a glass rod, then in turn add drops of sodium nitrite solution, sulphamic acid and *N*-1-naphthyl ethylene diamine, pausing between each. As before, the magenta colour forms slowly. The test is sensitive enough to detect benzodiazepine drugs in urine following normal therapeutic dosage, but it is not, of course, specific as it is given by any compound with a primary arylamino group which can be extracted under these conditions. In particular, phenylbutazone gives the test. This compound is hydrolysed by boiling hydrochloric acid to hydrazobenzene, which changes to benzidine. It can, however, be distinguished from the benzodiazepines by extracting the urine under acid conditions, using the method described above but substituting 1 ml. of dilute sulphuric acid for the borax, and re-extracting the chloroform with an alkaline spot. After drying, the spot is treated with ammonium vanadate solution, again dried, and then treated with concentrated sulphuric acid. Phenylbutazone gives a deep purple, but the benzodiazepines give no colour.

Acknowledgements: I wish to express my gratitude to Dr. Alan Gardner, Dr. M. Mitchenson, and Mr. J. V. J. Jackson for providing me with experimental material; to Messrs. Carlo Erba and Messrs. Roche Products Ltd. for generous gifts of the benzodiazepine drugs and their metabolites; and to Mrs. Frances Desmond for technical assistance.

REFERENCES

BADEN, M. M., VALANJU, N. N., VERMA, S. K., and VALANJU, S. N. (1972), Confirmed identification of biotransformed drugs in urine, *Am. J. clin. Path.*, **57**, 43–51.

BASTOS, M. L., KANANEN, G. E., YOUNG, R. M., MONTFORTE, J. R., and SUNSHINE, I. (1970), Detection of basic organic drugs and their metabolites in urine, *Clin. Chem.*, **16**, 931–940.

BECKETT, A. H., TUCKER, G. T., and MOFFAT, A. C. (1967), Routine detection and identification in urine of stimulants and other drugs, some of which may be used to modify performance in sport, *J. Pharm. Pharmac.*, **19**, 273–294.

BERRY, D. J., GROVE, J., WIDDOP, B., and WILLIS, J. H. P. (1970), The detection of drugs of dependence in urine, *Bull. Narcot.* **22**, 31–37.

BOWEN, D. A. L., GURR, D. M., and OPPENHEIM, G. B. (1970), Thin layer chromatographic laboratory analysis in cases from a drug addiction centre, *Clin. Toxicol.*, **3**, 89–95.

BRATTON, A. C. and MARSHALL, E. K. (1939), A new coupling component for sulphanilamide determination, *J. biol. Chem.*, **128**, 537–550.

BROICH, J. B., HOFFMAN, D. B., ANDRYAUSKAS, S., GALANTE, L., and UMBERGER, C. J. (1971), An improved method for rapid large-scale thin layer chromatographic urine screening for drugs of abuse, *J. Chromatog.*, **60**, 95–101.

CLARKE, E. G. C. (1971), Rapid detection of certain basic drugs in urine, *Br. med. J.*, **4**, 35–37.

DAVIDOW, B., PETRI, N. L., and QUAME, B. (1968), A thin-layer chromatographic screening procedure for detecting drug abuse, *Am. J. clin. Path.*, **50**, 714–719.

DOLE, V. P., CROWTHER, A., JOHNSON, J., MONSALVATGE, M., BILLER, B., and NELSON, S. S. (1972), Detection of narcotic, sedative and amphetamine drugs in urine, *N.Y.St. J. Med.*, **72**, 471–476.

DOLE, V. P., KIM, W. K., and EGLITIS, I. (1966), Detection of narcotic durgs, tranquillizers, amphetamines and barbiturates in urine, *J. Am. med. Ass.*, **198**, 115–118.

GARRIOTT, J. C., and STOLMAN, A. (1971), Detection of some psychotherapeutic drugs, *Clin. Toxicol.*, **4**, 225–243.

HO, I. K., LOH, H. H., and WAY, E. L. (1972), Mini thin-layer chromatography in the detection of narcotics in urine from subjects on a methadone maintenance program, *J. Chromatog.*, **65**, 577–579.

KOECHLIN, B. A., and D'ARCONTE, L. (1963), Determination of chlordiazepoxide (Librium) and of a metabolite of lactam character in plasma of humans, dogs and rats by a specific spectrophotometric micro method, *Analyt. Biochem.*, **5**, 195–207.

—, SCHWARTZ, M. A., KROL, G., and OBERHANSLI, W. (1965), The metabolic fate of C^{14}-labelled chlordiazepoxide in man, in the dog, and in the rat, *J. Pharmac. exp. Therap.*, **148**, 399–411.

MARKS, V., FRY, D., CHAPPLE, P. A. L., and GRAY, G. (1969), Application of urine analysis to diagnosis and treatment of heroin addiction, *Br. med. J.*, **2**, 153–155.

MORGAN, P. J. (1959), A method for the rapid detection of small concentrations of organic bases in urine, *Analyst*, **84**, 418–422.

MOSS, D. G. (1954), The estimation of butazolidin in blood, *J. clin. Path.*, 7, 344–347.

MULÉ, S. J. (1969), Identification of narcotics, barbiturates, amphetamines, tranquillizers and psychotomimetics in human urine, *J. Chromatog.*, **39**, 302–311.

ONO, M., ENGELKE, B. F., and FULTON, C. (1969), Procedures for assured identification of morphine, dihydromorphine, codeine, norcodeine, methadone, quinine, methamphetamine, etc. in human urine, *Bull. Narcot.*, **21**(2), 31–40.

PELZER, H., and MAASS, D. (1969), Pharmakokinetik und Metabolismus von 7-chlor-1, 3-dihydro-3-hydroxy-5-phenyl-2H-1, 4-benzodiazepin-2-on und dessen Hemisuccinat beim Menschen, *Arzneimittel-Forsch.*, **19**, 1652–1656.

PRIBILLA, O. (1965), Zum chemischen Nachweis von 1,3-Dihydro-7-nitro-5-phenyl-2H-1, 4-benzodiazepin-2-on, *Ibid.*, **15**, 1148–1152.

RAMSEY, J. and CAMPBELL, D. B. (1971), An ultra rapid method for the extraction of drugs from biological fluids, *J. Chromatog.*, **63**, 303–308.

REIDER, J. (1965), Methoden zür Bestimmung von 1,3-dihydro-7-nitro-5-phenyl-2H-1, 4-benzodiazepin-2-on und sienem Haupt metaboliten in biologischen. Proben und Ergebnisse von versuchen über die Pharmakokinetik und die Metabolismus dieser Substanz bei Mensch und Ratte, *Arzneimittel-Forsch.*, **15**, 1134–1148.

DE SILVA, J. A. F., KOECHLIN, B. A., and BADER, G. (1966), Blood level distribution patterns of diazepam and its major metabolites in man, *J. pharm. Sci.*, **55**, 692–702.

—, and PUGLIZI, C. V. (1970), Determination of medazepam (Nobrium), diazepam (Valium) and their major biotransformation products in blood and urine by election capture gas-liquid chromatography, *Ann. Chem.*, **42**, 1725–1736.

SCHWARTZ, M. A., and CARBONE, T. J. (1970), Metabolism of C^{14} medazepam hydrochloride in dog, rat, and man, *Biochem. Pharmac.*, **19**, 343–361.

—, KOECHLIN, B. A., POSTMA, E., PALMA, S., and KROL, G. (1965), Metabolism of diazepam in rat, dog and man. *J. Pharmac. exp. Therap.*, **149**, 423–435.

STEEL, J. W., BOLAN, M., and EYOLFSON, J. K. (1970), An improved method for detection of some stimulants, antihistamines and local anaesthetics in urine from athletes, *Can. J. pharm. Sci.* **5**, 107–111.
THÖMPSETT, S. L. (1968), Nitrazepam (Mogadon) in blood, serum and urine and Librium in urine, *J. clin. Path.*, **21**, 366–371.
WALKENSTEIN, S. S., WISER, R., GUDMUNDSEN, C. H., KIMMEL, H. B., and CORRADINO, R. A. (1964), Absorption, metabolism, and excretion of oxazepam and its succinate half-ester, *J. pharm. Sci.*, **53**, 1181–1186.
WEIST, F. R. (1968), Zum nachweis von 7-chlor-1, 3-dihydro-3-hydroxy-5-phenyl-2H-1, 4-benzodiazepin-2-on in biologischen Flussigkeiten, *Arzneimittel-Forsch.*, **18**, 87–89.

Post-mortem Diagnosis of Barbiturate Poisoning

D. J. GEE, R. A. DALLEY, M. A. GREEN, and L. A. PERKIN

Department of Forensic Medicine, University of Leeds

At the present time barbiturate poisoning must still rate as one of the most common causes of fatal poisoning. Thus, the Registrar General's figures for 1969 show that there were 1969 poisonings by sedatives and hypnotics, the group which includes barbiturates. In 1970, barbiturates alone accounted for about 1600 fatal poisonings.

This paper is meant to present barbiturate poisoning from the viewpoint of the forensic pathologist, performing the post mortem and puzzling over the cause of death. Also in an article on the liver/blood ratio in cases of barbiturate poisoning, Curry and Sunshine (1960) stated that a systematic analysis of heart blood and femoral blood in a large number of cases would be desirable. This is, in part, what we and other members of our department, from time to time, have endeavoured to do over a period of several years.

The period of time covered by this survey is 7 years, from 1963 to 1969. The cases are all what might be called standard coroners' cases of death from barbiturate poisoning occurring outside hospital. We have no data on treated or non-fatal cases. The number of poisonings seen during the 7-year period was 202. The total number of autopsies performed during that period by the department was 6200, so that

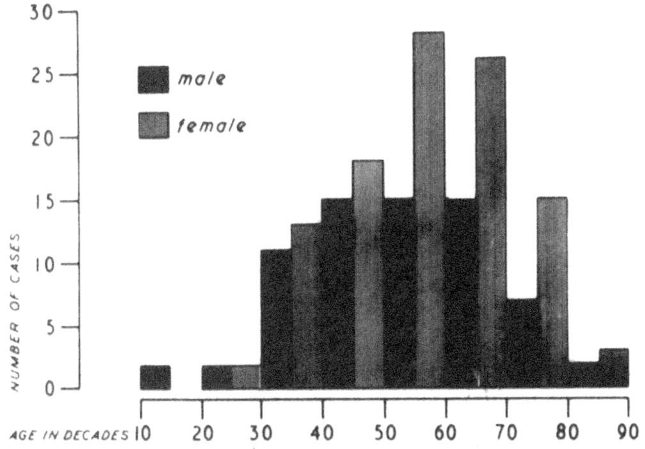

Fig. 1. Number of barbiturate poisonings, by sex and age, seen over a seven-year period (1963–9) in the Department of Forensic Medicine, University of Leeds.

death from barbiturate poisoning represents some 3–4 per cent of our autopsy practice.

The general characteristics of our series are similar, I would think, to that of many others. Thus women outnumber men – there being 81 men to 121 women, a ratio of 2:3. The age distribution, shown in *Fig.* 1, is in some respects curious, with men showing no significant peak, while women appear to die from this cause mainly between the ages of 50 and 70. Whether this is related to involutional physiological states, to bereavement, or to some other factor, we do not know.

The types of barbiturate causing fatal poisoning are shown in *Table* 1. One

Table 1. Types of barbiturates causing fatal poisoning in the 202 cases seen in the Department of Forensic Medicine, University of Leeds.

Drug taken	*No. of cases*
Tuinal (amylobarbitone and quinalbarbitone)	74
Amytal (amylobarbitone)	34
Nembutal (pentobarbitone)	25
Soneryl (butobarbitone)	12
Seconal (quinalbarbitone)	7
Barbiturate and alcohol	34
Mixed drugs	16

striking feature is the popularity of Tuinal, and another is the total absence from our series of the long-acting barbiturates, such as phenobarbitone. A reasonable explanation is that persons taking long-acting drugs did not die quickly, and so reached hospital and escaped our attentions. However, since quite a few of the persons in our series were not found for several days after last being seen alive, it is still surprising that we did not encounter any phenobarbitone poisonings.

The approximate proportions of the different barbiturates remained much the same throughout the period, Tuinal always being the most common, followed by Amytal, with Nembutal close to it and others trailing very far behind.

Comparatively few of our cases took alcohol at the same time as the barbiturates, and fewer still took a mixture of drugs, either a mixture of barbiturates, or of a barbiturate and either a tranquillizer, a salicylate, or carbon monoxide. We have excluded the cases involving alcohol and other drugs from the subsequent discussion of tissue levels because we cannot be sure what allowance to make for the other substances.

Before one starts to think about analyses and tissue levels, one has, quite obviously, to appreciate that the death that one is dealing with is probably due to barbiturate poisoning. For the morbid anatomists, rather than the analysts, this is one aspect of the subject which we feel keenly, because we are constantly oppressed by the fear, in performing almost any autopsy, unless we trip over the hatchet sticking out of the man's head, of missing a death by poisoning, because of our lack of suspicion, or because of the lack of any suggestive signs at autopsy and the presence of sufficient other explanation for death, such as coronary artery disease, to allay any anxieties which we might have.

In fact, of our 202 cases, in all but 24 the diagnosis was suggested by the information supplied by the Coroner's Officer or the police before the autopsy commenced – the past history of suicide attempts, the empty pill bottle beside the bed, and so on. Of the remaining 24 cases, although the story of the circumstances of the death had nothing in it to suggest poisoning, in 14 cases the autopsy findings were characteristic, or at least suspicious.

In my experience it is comparatively rare to find tablet traces on the body surface and exceedingly rare to find the blisters which others find such a characteristic feature. However, internally, the thickened, dark red-brown oesophagus, sometimes filled with a coloured jelly, and a congested, mildly corroded stomach are fairly frequent features, as shown in *Figs.* 2 and 3. Nevertheless these features may also, of

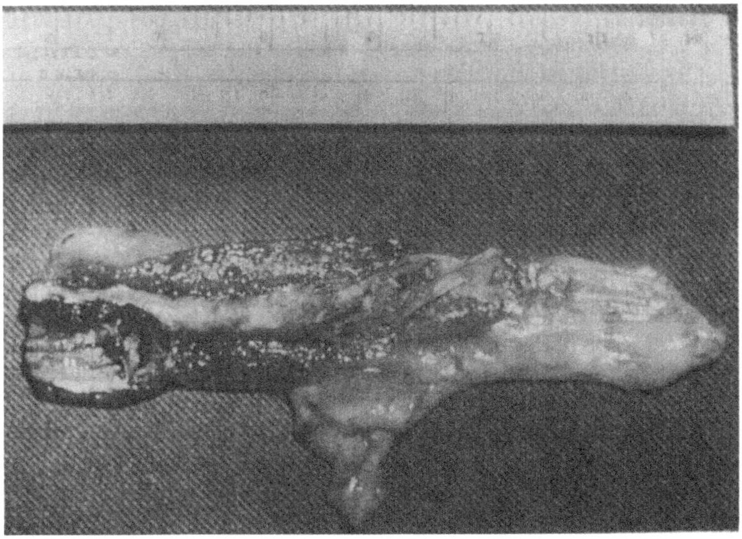

Fig. 2. Thickened, discoloured oesophagus containing a plug of coloured (blue) jelly-like material in a case of barbiturate poisoning.

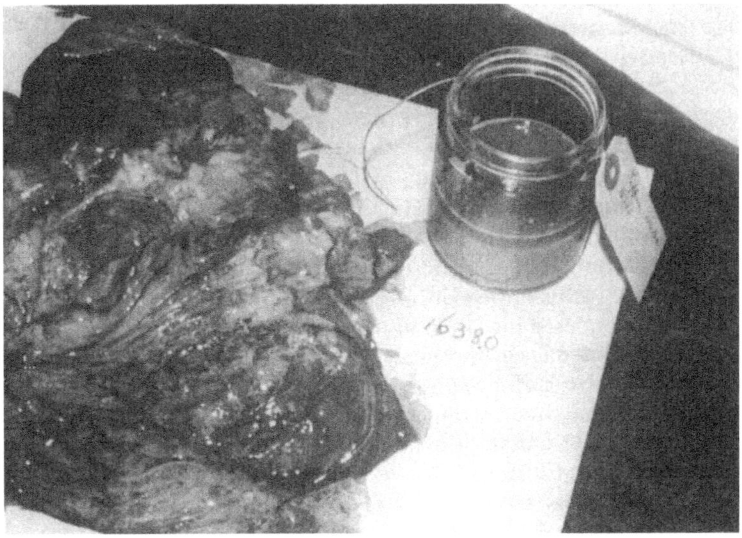

Fig. 3. Stomach from a case of barbiturate poisoning, showing congestion and slight corrosion of the mucosa.

course, be absent, and in 10 of our cases (5 per cent), which we would submit is a not insignificant number, there were neither history nor autopsy findings to indicate poisoning. The fact that they were picked up is due largely to the practice in our department of screening a blood sample from almost every case by the method devised by Curry (1963), using a small beaker on a mechanical stirrer, with extraction of the blood by chloroform, and subsequent additions of a mercury solution and dithizone reagent. We have found this method very valuable as a preliminary sorting test in routine autopsy practice.

We have encountered false positive results only very infrequently, but when they occur we have found them almost always due either to the fact that the deceased was an elderly diabetic on an oral hypoglycaemic agent, such as tolbutamide, or else that early putrefactive changes have occurred and presumably liberated free fatty acids into the blood.

Perhaps 10 cases, only a little over one case a year, of barbiturate poisoning which would otherwise pass to the grave totally undetected, is not an alarmingly high figure to report from one practice, but in 7 years that equals 1·4 cases per year. Since we do about 1000 autopsies a year that is an incidence of about 0·1 per cent of deaths reported to the Coroner in our area. Since the annual death rate in this country at present is about 500,000, one could speculate, and of course it is no more than speculation and may be quite wrong, that about 500 deaths could occur each year from barbiturate poisoning and be totally undetected. If one were to continue to speculate about how many similar deaths there could be from other commonly available medicinal drugs, such as the tranquillizers and antidepressants, then the whole situation becomes infinitely more complicated, but this is to digress too far into the realms of pure speculation.

What is, of course, undeniable in the experience of anyone having much to do with the post-mortem investigation of barbiturate deaths, is the remarkable way in which the circumstances of these deaths may be misleading to the investigator, or the apparently almost incredible lack of awareness of other persons around the intending suicide of what he or she is doing. For instance, one of the oddest and potentially most dangerous or disastrous of all our cases concerned a boy of 15 who had a girl friend with whom he had a row one day. In the evening he went into town with another lad and chanced to meet his erstwhile girl friend with a new paramour and a group of friends. Inevitably words followed, then a scuffle, and in the course of this the boy was knocked down, striking his head, and later some said that he was kicked while on the ground. Then the fighting stopped and the lad, assisted by his friend, got up and set off home rather disconsolately. His parents were out that evening but arrived home shortly, probably a matter of ten minutes or so, after him. Hearing the story and finding him rather shaken and a little dizzy they put him to bed with a hot-water bottle to sleep it off, and the reassuring sound in the morning, when his father looked in, of deep stertorous breathing, indicated that the desired result was being achieved. Only when at about midday he was found not to be breathing at all did it appear that all was far from well.

At autopsy the police were treating this death as a potential case of manslaughter. The post-mortem did not reveal the expected fractured skull or intracranial haematoma, only a large bruise at the back of the scalp and pronounced cerebral oedema, but further enquiries elicited the fact that the boy had, on at least two previous occasions, suffered head injuries of a comparatively minor nature which were succeeded by severe and prolonged concussion, and so we thought it probable that he was one of those odd persons with an unstable cerebrovascular system and had died from respiratory depression from cerebral oedema. Only because he was a teenager and we thought might have been taking pep pills or amphetamines, did we think it wise to analyse for some of the commoner drugs of minor addiction, and were startled to discover the presence of a fatal dose of Amytal. Further enquiries revealed the presence in the house of a large number of ½-grain Amytal tablets which had been prescribed for his father at some time in the past. It then became obvious that on returning home, having lost both his fight and his girl friend in one day, and with his parents absent, he took a good handful of these tablets, equivalent to 43 grains, obviously with suicidal intent. His opponent in the scuffle had a narrow escape from a criminal charge.

Given that the need for analysis for barbiturate has become apparent, either from history, autopsy findings, or screening tests, the analysis has been performed in the Department of the Leeds City Analyst. Samples normally used consisted of peripheral blood, derived from the femoral vein, liver, brain, stomach contents and, where available, urine. Out of our 202 cases about 80 right heart blood levels have also been estimated.

The methods of analysis for barbiturate used have been those of Broughton (1956), using ultra violet spectrophotometry. The stomach contents are extracted with ether from acid solution and the sodium hydroxide fraction assayed by the method of Broughton. The total amount of barbiturate was determined, no distinction being made between the active drug and the metabolite.

From the average of the peripheral blood and brain tissue barbiturate levels, and the known body weight, an estimate of the amount of barbiturate circulating has been obtained using the Widmark factor of 0·7 for males and 0·6 for females. Then by addition of the amount of barbiturate remaining in the stomach the minimum total amount of drug taken has been estimated, though of course no allowance can be made for drug metabolized. The results of the series are given for Tuinal (*Table* 2), Amytal (*Table* 3), Nembutal (*Table* 4), Seconal (*Table* 5), and Soneryl (*Table* 6). In the case F.M. 13223, of poisoning by Tuinal (*Table* 2), we cannot exclude contamination as the cause of the remarkably high blood level, and this case was not included when calculating average levels (*Table* 7).

It seems to us to be worthy of comment that so few mortuaries in which autopsies on these types of cases are usually performed are equipped with means of obtaining the weight of the body. In the old Leeds City Mortuary there was a type of body-weighing machine, on which almost all these calculations in this series are based – one of the few good features in a mortuary of otherwise quite unbelievably Dickensian squalor. The new public mortuary which the City has built has a specially constructed weighbridge, corrected for the weight of the trolley on which the body is lying, and all bodies, once undressed, measured and temperatures recorded, are wheeled on to this platform and weighed. We cannot think of any other public mortuary we visit with facilities for weighing bodies, and with some notable exceptions, few hospital mortuaries have these facilities either. This means that for interpretation of the death one is relying solely on barbiturate levels in the tissues which one has taken, a procedure which we hope to show is not without difficulty.

One feature obviously missing from these tables and one which we have found it impossible to obtain with any degree of accuracy, is the length of time between consumption of the drug and death. From the very nature of the cases very often all that is known is that a person was last seen alive and apparently well by neighbours on one day, and was then found dead in bed the following day or possibly several days later, so that only the maximum time that could have been taken to die is

Table 2. Amount of barbiturate in stomach contents, blood, urine, and various tissues from 74 cases of fatal poisoning by Tuinal (amylobarbitone and quinalbarbitone)

Case number (F.M.No)	*Sex*	*Age*	*Barbiturate Level* Stomach contents (mg.)	Peripheral blood (mg. per 100 ml.)	Heart blood (mg. per 100 ml.)	Liver (mg. per 100 g.)	Brain (mg. per 100 g.)	Urine (mg. per 100 ml.)	*Total circulating barbiturate (mg.)*	*Total barbiturate taken (mg.)*
9,215	F.	–	–	1·7	4·7	20·7	4·2	–	960	–
9,225	F.	–	840	2·3	6·4	20·0	7·5	0·13	1800	2640
9,355	M.	32	48	2·7	3·2	3·0	2·7	2·5	1080	–
9,472	F.	67	1740	3·9	7·9	24·0	5·6	2·0	1500	3240
9,551	M.	–	4020	3·4	3·4	9·7	3·7	–	1740	5760
9,562	F.	71	120	5·6	6·3	7·2	6·5	–	2700	2820
9,746	F.	–	5040	–	4·5	15·6	2·6	–	1260	6300
9,947	F.	–	4380	3·0	–	14·0	4·7	–	1320	5700
10,033	F.	–	84	2·6	2·9	6·6	4·3	0·7	984	1068
10,112	F.	–	360	3·6	–	29·0	5·9	–	1420	1980
10,471	F.	46	60	3·4	–	14·5	3·1	–	1500	1560
10,548	F.	46	2760	5·0	–	10·8	4·1	–	1860	4620
10,692	F.	76	180	1·8	6·3	19·0	5·0	–	1500	1680
10,781	M.	51	–	1·8	2·0	8·0	1·7	4·2	1080	– *
10,794	F.	77	2208	1·0	–	12·6	2·8	–	756	2964*
10,876	M.	81	540	1·6	3·8	8·1	2·0	–	540	1080
10,900	M.	49	60	2·2	–	10·9	3·3	–	1380	1440*
10,906B	F.	39	1440	1·9	4·0	10·4	2·4	–	900	2340
10,948	F.	57	2700	2·2	8·8	18·0	5·5	–	1800	4500
10,990B	F.	46	2460	2·0	3·3	12·5	3·9	NIL	1020	3480
11,212	F.	58	180	5·8	–	9·6	5·1	–	1740	1920
11,242B	F.	77	2340	1·9	5·3	9·7	2·8	0·8	1440	3780
11,433	F.	71	660	2·0	6·4	14·0	5·5	–	2400	3060
11,468	F.	55	690	4·8	–	18·7	4·2	–	1710	2400*
11,489	F.	63	3000	2·9	–	15·0	2·9	1·0	1140	4140
11,564	F.	76	6600	3·5	–	37·0	7·3	–	2220	8820*
11,579A	F.	60	840	2·7	–	12·5	5·8	–	2580	3420
11,583	F.	74	840	4.2	–	11·0	5·2	–	1680	2520
11,584	M.	37	240	2·2	–	7·7	5·1	–	1860	2100
11,610B	M.	54	4440	5·1	–	28·0	6·4	–	2580	7020
11,670	M.	62	636	2·0	3·2	17·0	3·7	–	1266	1902
11,778	M.	59	120	6·4	–	22·0	7·0	–	3120	3240
11,813	F.	65	180	3·7	–	12·0	4·3	–	1440	1620
11,987	F.	71	NIL	1·8	–	3·2	2·5	5·1	720	–
12,015	F.	49	2070	12·1	–	39·4	9·1	–	2910	4980

Case number (F.M.No)	Sex	Age	Barbiturate Level: Stomach contents (mg.)	Peripheral blood (mg. per 100 ml.)	Heart blood (mg. per 100 ml.)	Liver (mg. per 100 g.)	Brain (mg. per 100 g.)	Urine (mg. per 100 ml.)	Total circulating barbiturate (mg.)	Total barbiturate taken (mg.)
12,098B	F.	72	1488	4·5	–	24·0	4·9	–	1080	2568
12,107	F.	36	1500	3·2	–	14·0	4·6	–	1860	3360
12,186A	F.	52	2520	2·5	–	19·0	2·9	–	1800	4320
12,188B	F.	67	NIL	1·3	–	4·1	2·5	–	720	–
12,193	F.	63	1680	3·9	–	20·0	5·7	–	1380	3060
12,234	F.	61	4380	3·7	–	29·0	6·3	–	1620	6000
12,244	F.	43	1680	3·6	–	12·7	4·9	–	1380	3060*
12,272	M.	52	–	1·2	–	5·5	2·5	–	780	–
12,312	F.	55	3120	5·2	7·1	39·0	9·5	3·7	2160	5280
12,358	F.	–	3780	3·1	4·0	44·0	6·4	–	1800	5580
12,400	M.	68	3	2·5	–	6·2	3·5	–	1200	–
12,434A	M.	75	3840	3·6	–	22·0	4·8	–	1920	5760
12,441A	F.	35	1656	4·8	–	21·4	7·7	–	2190	3840
12,494	F.	52	–	2·0	–	2·5	3·0	–	550	–
12,522	F.	64	3100	2·0	4·6	14·0	8·1	1·5	1800	4900
12,612	F.	34	4500	5·1	5·4	17·0	8·9	3·4	1620	6120
12,746	M.	44	360	2·0	2·8	11·4	4·8	–	2280	2640*
12,806	M.	36	1020	2·1	5·4	23·0	4·3	2·2	1860	2880
13,038	M.	76	1260	2·5	4·2	20·0	6·6	1·2	1620	2880
13,093B	F.	66	880	6·4	–	30·0	6·2	1·7	2330	3210
13,096	F.	57	420	2·0	4·6	26·0	6·5	–	1560	1980
13,104	F.	42	60	2·0	1·8	6·8	3·7	–	1020	1080
13,143	F.	73	1800	4·2	2·9	16·0	3·8	0·5	1260	3060
13,169	F.	59	63	2·5	5·0	26·0	9·3	39·0	2220	2280*
13,223	F.	50	2880	29·0	–	34·0	7·6	–	3060	5940
13,273	M.	33	180	2·1	–	10·0	3·8	–	1260	1440
13,365	M.	49	3000	5·2	–	17·0	6·5	2·0	3840	6840
13,570	M.	50	2800	0·9	–	18·0	4·4	–	2600	5400
13,603	F.	62	91	2·1	–	9·4	4·4	1·6	1980	2100
13,612	F.	31	90	3·3	–	8·5	6·2	6·0	1020	1110
13,674	F.	69	4000	2·1	5·4	26·0	9·0	–	1400	5400*
13,929	F.	68	1200	2·0	–	15·4	4·8	0·5	970	2170*
13,987	F.	60	1260	1·4	–	29·1	5·2	–	1210	2470
14,044	M.	30	650	1·4	–	6·4	3·0	0·9	1300	2000
14,136	F.	65	800	2·0	–	27·0	4·7	–	1230	2030*
14,128	F.	46	–	1·4	–	3·6	1·2	2·5	360	–
14,192	M.	85	1700	2·5	3·3	16·8	6·4	3·1	1530	3230
14,272	F.	53	1780	2·0	5·3	23·0	7·4	4·4	1510	3290*
14,387	F.	50	2200	2·4	–	12·0	6·8	9·0	1500	3700

*Died within 4 hours of taking the drug.

Table 3. Amount of barbiturate in stomach contents, blood, urine, and various tissues from 34 cases of fatal poisoning by Amytal (amylobarbitone)

Case number (F.M.No)	*Sex*	*Age*	*Barbiturate Level* Stomach contents (mg.)	Peripheral blood (mg. per 100 ml.)	Heart blood (mg. per 100 ml.)	Liver (mg. per 100 g.)	Brain (mg. per 100 g.)	Urine (mg. per 100 ml.)	*Total circulating barbiturate (mg.)*	*Total barbiturate taken (mg.)*
9,024	M.	–	444	2·9	–	11·1	–	–	1320	1764
9,195	M.	–	420	5·1	7·6	17·8	–	–	1920	2340
9,275	F.	–	100	4·2	6·9	20·5	8·7	–	1440	1530
9,465	M.	70	600	4·5	–	16·1	–	3·2	1980	2580
9,703	F.	–	2280	3·4	3·8	5·2	3·4	–	960	3240
10,049	F.	86	1500	3·6	6·2	8·0	5·1	–	1380	2880
10,331	F.	26	420	4·3	–	5·6	4·5	1·8	1260	1680*
10,574	F.	59	2880	3·4	4·8	7·3	3·3	–	1440	4320*
10,697	F.	53	3900	7·0	8·2	16·0	6·5	–	3120	7020
10,718	F.	54	780	2·6	2·8	3·9	2·6	–	900	1680
11,307	F.	30	2460	8·9	–	31·0	–	–	3540	6000*
11,606	M.	37	1440	4·7	–	6·7	4·6	–	2880	4320
11,626	F.	35	180	3·7	–	17·0	6·8	–	1740	1920
11,777	M.	64	360	1·8	–	4·5	2·0	–	720	1080
11,818	F.	42	9840	7·8	–	18·0	11·0	–	3300	12780
11,817	F.	47	360	2·8	–	11·0	2·6	–	900	1260
11,803	F.	40	NIL	1·3	–	4·6	2·9	–	660	–
12,457	M.	43	6480	5·8	–	14·7	–	26·9	3180	9660
12,554	F.	63	2280	5·3	5·8	2·3	8·6	6·2	1920	4200
12,572	F.	58	6	2·5	–	2·4	2·3	–	480	540
12,613	F.	53	12	2·7	2·0	5·9	2·8	5·9	900	–
12,808	M.	15	1080	3·2	3·7	8·5	–	1·8	1500	2580
12,841	F.	73	4500	2·5	–	22·0	7·3	–	2160	6660
13,120	M.	68	–	1·2	–	2·1	2·8	–	1080	–
13,209	F.	47	360	2·3	4·5	23·0	12·0	0·9	2520	2880*
13,592	M.	66	1350	2·1	2·2	14·0	5·8	–	2600	3950
13,704	F.	65	800	3·3	13·8	42·0	9·7	–	1800	2600
13,891	M.	53	1750	5·7	5·3	14·7	7·7	16·3	2870	4620
13,952	M.	67	–	4·9	–	5·3	3·6	–	2060	–
14,004	M.	43	2470	2·9	2·8	7·9	4·4	2·4	2000	4470
14,162	F.	39	830	4·1	–	29·0	7·8	–	1690	2520
14,230	M.	67	570	3·3	–	8·3	2·7	1·4	1110	1680
14,297	F.	70	–	3·8	–	17·0	10·0	–	1900	–
14,371	F.	68	900	1·7	6·7	26·0	6·6	–	1700	2600

*Died within 4 hours of taking the drug.

Table 4. Amount of barbiturate in stomach contents, blood, urine, and various tissues from 25 cases of fatal poisoning by Nembutal (pentobarbitone).

Case number (F.M.No)	*Sex*	*Age*	*Barbiturate Level* Stomach contents (mg.)	Peripheral blood (mg. per 100 ml.)	Heart blood (mg. per 100 ml.)	Liver (mg. per 100 g.)	Brain (mg. per 100 g.)	Urine (mg. per 100 ml.)	*Total circulating barbiturate (mg.)*	*Total barbiturate taken (mg.)*
9,092	F.	65	108	1·3	–	2·1	1·6	–	330	510
9,106	F.	36	2220	1·0	5·1	16·6	5·3	–	1020	3240
10,025	F.	–	522	2·5	7·1	25·0	5·8	1·5	1638	2160
10,783	M.	58	804	4·1	7·0	14·5	2·8	–	2022	2820*
11,083	F.	54	720	8·3	–	24·0	–	–	2760	3480*
11,207	M.	67	360	3·1	6·7	4·9	–	–	1500	1860
11,259	F.	67	–	2·5	–	7·0	2·5	–	1200	–
11,305	F.	75	300	3·9	–	12·0	–	–	1200	1500
11,431	F.	53	780	3·0	5·9	24·0	4·4	–	1860	2640
11,534A	M.	40	1080	3·5	–	8·8	5·9	–	1980	3060
11,712	M.	46	3180	2·2	–	12·7	4·3	–	1440	4620
11,967	F.	42	780	1·5	–	–	–	–	480	1260
11,969	F.	35	360	1·9	4·9	9·4	5·9	–	1380	1740
12,058C	F.	61	360	5·4	–	15·0	9·4	3·8	2520	2880
12,934	M.	62	3960	6·0	14·6	20·0	8·0	1·6	3360	7320
12,137	M.	38	2460	6·5	–	15·5	5·1	–	3060	5520
12,144C	M.	58	4878	3·8	–	30·3	6·6	NIL	2178	7056
12,313	F.	54	126	4·0	4·6	14·6	4·8	–	1560	1686
12,328	M.	76	60	2·1	4·9	24·0	4·4	–	1740	1800
12,363	F.	43	NIL	1·9	2·2	5·1	2·9	–	840	–
12,624	F.	64	70	3·1	4·6	27·0	6·6	2·3	1380	1440
12,755	M.	40	2920	2·3	2·3	11·0	3·6	–	1550	4570
12,911	F.	69	3780	1·9	4·8	23·0	6·0	2·6	1620	5400
13,115	F.	80	6	1·5	–	3·8	1·4	–	–	–
13,097	F.	59	–	4·0	–	8·3	5·8	–	1680	–

*Died within 4 hours of taking drug.

Table 5. Amount of barbiturate in stomach contents, blood, urine, and various tissues from 7 cases of fatal poisoning by Seconal (quinalbarbitone).

Case number (F.M.No)	Sex	Age	Barbiturate Level: Stomach contents (mg.)	Peripheral blood (mg. per 100 ml.)	Heart blood (mg. per 100 ml.)	Liver (mg. per 100 g.)	Brain (mg. per 100 g.)	Urine (mg. per 100 ml.)	*Total circulating barbiturate (mg.)*	*Total barbiturate taken (mg.)*
9,027	F.	38	390	2·7	–	9·0	–	–	960	1350
9,899	M.	–	720	1·6	2·5	3·9	1·6	–	540	1260
10,883	M.	32	660	2·4	3·2	6·4	3·3	–	1260	1920
11,425	F.	36	6	1·4	–	3·4	1·4	–	–	– ★
11,723	M.	40	15	1·1	–	3·5	1·8	1·3	840	–
12,007	F.	48	NIL	2·3	–	4·9	2·4	–	600	–
13,631	M.	68	–	1·5	–	6·3	3·8	–	880	–

★Died within 4 hours of taking the drug.

Table 6. Amount of barbiturate in stomach contents, blood, urine, and various tissues from 12 cases of fatal poisoning by Soneryl (butobarbitone).

Case number (F.M.No)	Sex	Age	Barbiturate Level: Stomach contents (mg.)	Peripheral blood (mg. per 100 ml.)	Heart blood (mg. per 100 ml.)	Liver (mg. per 100 g.)	Brain (mg. per 100 g.)	Urine (mg. per 100 ml.)	*Total circulating barbiturate (mg.)*	*Total barbiturate taken (mg.)*
9,069	M.	50	600	5·5	7·5	16·6	–	–	2640	3240
9,251	M.	–	96	2·7	3·0	5·2	3·5	–	1260	1356
9,380	M.	–	2460	1·1	–	4·9	2·1	–	960	3420
10,227	F.	–	NIL	5·5	–	6·9	5·5	–	1560	–
10,344	M.	28	300	10·2	11·0	14·8	12·0	7·0	3480	3780
11,155	F.	46	NIL	4·5	5·7	6·7	3·9	9·4	1500	–
11,728	M.	50	180	6·0	–	8·3	4·6	–	2460	2640
12,039	F.	53	162	5·0	–	10·9	4·3	–	1332	1494
13,375	F.	–	6000	1·6	3·4	12·0.	4·7	–	1320	7320
13,399	F.	93	384	5·9	–	12·2	7·4	–	1422	1806★
13,468	F.	59	96	1·7	–	6·0	2·4	–	984	1080
14,086	M.	55	2050	5·6	–	11·5	7·7	–	2300	4350

★Died within 4 hours of taking the drug.

Table 7. Average levels of barbiturate in blood and tissues from all cases of the five barbiturate drugs encountered, together with average barbiturate levels in cases known to have died within four hours of taking the drug.

Drug	*Number of cases*	*Average barbiturate concentration* Peripheral blood (mg. per 100 ml.)	Heart blood (mg. per 100 ml.)	Liver (mg. per 100 g.)	Brain (mg. per 100 g.)
All cases					
Tuinal	74	3·0	4·6	16·8	5·0
Amytal	34	3·8	5·4	13·2	5·6
Nembutal	25	2·7	5·7	14·9	5·0
Soneryl	12	5·2	6·1	9·6	5·3
Seconal	7	1·9	2·8	5·3	2·5
Dying within 4 hours					
Tuinal	12	2·5	4·1	19·1	5·4
Amytal	4	4·7	4·6	16·7	4·9
Nembutal	2	6·2	7·0	19·2	2·8

known. But in view of the well-known rapidity of action of some short-acting barbiturates, this type of information is of relatively little value. It is sometimes still not appreciated just how rapidly such fatalities may occur. Thus in one of our cases a man consumed a barbiturate and died from the effects within about 20 minutes while his wife went to the shops around the corner, and on another occasion a young woman swallowed her capsules standing at the kitchen sink looking down into the garden and must have died so rapidly that she virtually went into instantaneous rigor, since, according to the police description when found, she was still standing at the sink, though rather bent forward over the bowl.

However, the most meaningful attempt which we felt we should make to indicate the relation of tissue levels to rapidity of death was to separate off those cases in which it appeared the person must have died within 4 hours from those where the length of time taken could not be determined except within very wide limits. *Table* 7 gives the average tissue levels from all the cases of the five different barbiturate drugs encountered together with the levels in those cases known to have died within four hours of consuming the drug. Except in the case of Nembutal the levels are not significantly different from the main group of cases, but this would appear to bear the probably obvious conclusion that with these drugs, taken in such circumstances, without anyone else present, death occurs fairly rapidly, usually within a few hours, and that with such rapid deaths the level in the liver always tends to be high.

Given that in most of the cases we have no idea of how long it took the person to die, one tends to rely on the ratio between the different blood and tissue levels and of course the amount remaining unabsorbed in the stomach, though that last is a very unreliable feature. However, the ratios would appear to depend, to some extent at any rate, on the nature of the barbiturate taken. Thus *Table* 8 shows the ratios between the average levels in the various tissues for the different barbiturates. One reasonably constant feature does appear to be the ratio between the heart blood and the brain levels.

Table 8. Ratios between average barbiturate levels in various tissues for the five different barbiturate drugs encountered

Ratio of average barbiturate concentrations	*Barbiturate* Tuinal	Amytal	Nembutal	Soneryl	Seconal
Liver/peripheral blood	6/1	4/1	5/1	2/1	2·5/1
Liver/heart blood	4/1	2·5/1	2·5/1	2/1	2/1
Heart blood/peripheral blood	2/1	1/1	2/1	1/1	3/2
Brain/peripheral blood	2/1	3/2	2/1	1/1	1/1
Brain/heart blood	1/1	1/1	1/1	1/1	1/1
Brain/liver	1/3	1/2	1/3	1/2	1/2·5

Since one level to which one particularly pays attention is the ratio of blood to liver, we thought that it was of some interest to determine the ratio between the heart blood and peripheral blood levels to the liver level in five cases known to have died within four hours of taking the barbiturate (*Table* 9). The ratio of heart blood to liver remains almost constant, though there is a considerable range in the ratio between the peripheral blood and the liver. Obviously if one took either the one or the other ratio alone, in some of the cases one could reach totally different conclusions.

Table 9. Ratios of barbiturate in blood to that in liver in five cases which died within four hours of taking barbiturate (Tuinal)

Case number (F.M.No)	*Ratio* Peripheral blood/liver	Heart blood/liver
10,781	1/4	1/4
12,746	1/5	1/4
13,169	1/13	1/5
13,674	1/13	1/5
14,272	1/11	1/5

This result is due to the fact that on the whole the heart blood level appears to be directly related to the tissue levels, in particular to the brain level, and rises with increase in the liver level, while in general the peripheral blood level remains constant, even though the other levels are rising. This is demonstrated in *Fig.* 4. As the amount of barbiturate in the liver increases, so do the amounts in the heart blood and the brain, but there is scarcely any change in the peripheral blood level. This seems to fit in with the fact that blood levels reported in cases treated in hospital are usually very much higher than those found in persons dying at home, and that it is common for persons dying rapidly from barbiturate poisoning at home to have blood levels of the order of 2 mg. per 100 ml., more or less constantly. In fact, then, peripheral blood levels from common barbiturate poisonings seem to be almost always at about the 2–3 mg. per 100 ml. level irrespective of other tissue levels.

It occurred to us that the discrepancy between the levels in the heart and the peripheral blood could, in fact, be due to an artefact similar to those described as affecting the levels of alcohol and sugar in heart bloods, caused either by movement

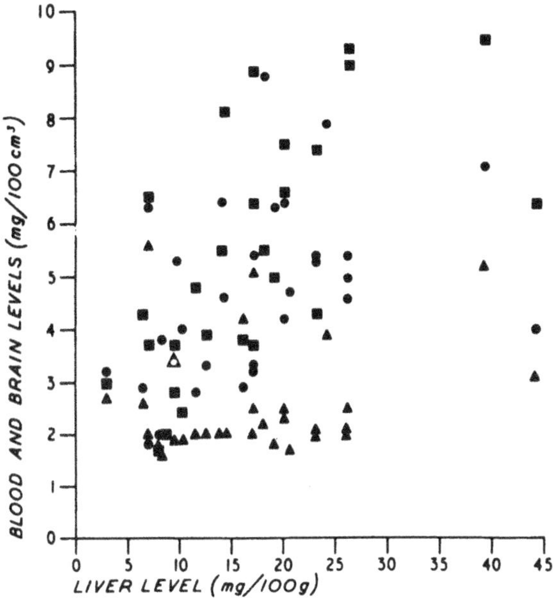

Fig. 4. Relationship between levels of barbiturate (Tuinal) in liver with those in brain (■), heart blood (●), and peripheral blood (▲).

of blood to or from the heart during the period of time after death, or by diffusion from the stomach. In fact we found, from the figures for poisoning for one year, that there appeared to be no constant increase in the heart blood level with increasing time after death.

Regarding the possibility of diffusion from the liver or from the stomach we could find no constant relationship between the level of barbiturate in the heart blood and that remaining in the stomach. In order to exclude the possibility of direct diffusion from the liver, in three cases we estimated the amount of barbiturate in the blood from the left side of the heart, as well as that from the right (*Table* 10).

Table 10. Barbiturate levels in blood from peripheral vein and left and right sides of the heart in three cases of barbiturate poisoning.

Case number (F.M.No)	*Drug*	*Barbiturate concentration (mg. per 100 ml.)* Peripheral blood	Right heart blood	Left heart blood
13,096	Tuinal	2·0	4·6	5·0
13,209	Amytal	2·3	4·8	4·2
13,038	Tuinal	2·5	4·2	4·9

The reasonably close similarity between the left and right heart barbiturate levels appears to be sufficient to exclude diffusion as a factor.

The alternative explanation for the higher heart blood level is that it represents an admixture with blood from the alimentary circulation rich in freshly absorbed barbiturate. We attempted to confirm this by assuming, on the authority of physiological textbooks, that the blood in the right atrium is derived equally from the superior and inferior vena cavae, and that of the blood entering the heart from the inferior vena cava, roughly half is derived from the liver. If the liver tissue level of barbiturate were the same as that of the blood passing through it from the portal circulation and the levels of barbiturate in the peripheral blood and liver tissue were known, one could attempt to calculate what the heart blood level should be. *Table* 11 represents the results of some calculations on this basis and a comparison of the calculated and actual heart blood levels. The orders are roughly right, and in some cases are very close, but if anything the actual blood level is slightly lower than the calculated level, suggesting that the liver level is not just the level of the blood flowing through it, but, as one might expect, some is actually stored in the tissue out of circulation. This is in agreement with the findings of Moghrabi and Curry (1970).

Table 11. Comparison of calculated and actual (measured) levels of barbiturate in heart blood.

Case number (F.M.No)	*Barbiturate concentration* Peripheral blood (mg. per 100 ml.)	Liver (mg. per 100 g.)	Theoretical heart blood (mg. per 100 ml.)	Actual heart blood (mg. per 100 ml.)
13,209	2·3	23·0	7·0	4·8
12,843	6·8	24·0	11·1	11·2
13,169	2·5	26·0	8·4	5·7
13,096	2·0	26·0	8·0	4·8
12,911	1·9	23·0	7·0	4·8
12,806	2·1	23·0	7·3	5·4
13,038	2·5	20·0	6·9	4·2
13,375	1·6	12·0	4·2	3·4
12,746	2·0	11·4	4·3	2·8
12,755	2·3	11·0	4·5	2·3
12,808	3·2	8·5	4·5	3·7
13,104	2·0	6·8	3·2	1·8

Thus it seems likely that the various tissue levels represent:

1. Barbiturate remaining in the stomach.
2. Barbiturate passing through and stored in the liver.
3. That the right heart blood barbiturate level is a true blood level derived from the mixture of blood from the liver and the general circulation. This level of barbiturate is distributed via the left heart to the tissues.
4. That tissues, such as the brain, with a high lipoid content and a large share of the circulation rapidly accumulate a level equivalent to that in the blood reaching them.
5. That blood returning from the tissues contains barbiturate which tends to remain at a fairly low constant level until again replenished from the alimentary circulation.

Our results appear to indicate that:

a. It is important, for the interpretation of analytical results, always to know where the blood sample came from.

b. A sample of heart blood is probably a better indication of the amount of barbiturate circulating than is one of peripheral blood.

c. Relatively constant peripheral blood levels may indicate some phenomenon such as protein binding, but this needs further investigation.

d. The diagnosis of barbiturate poisoning, even nowadays, is not foolproof as far as the pathologist is concerned.

Acknowledgements: The authors would like to acknowledge their indebtedness to Professor C. J. Polson who was Head of the Department of Forensic Medicine during the period of this survey, to Mr. P. B. Gaunt who was responsible for carrying out the screening tests, to Miss R. Bailey who prepared many of the charts and diagrams, and to Her Majesty's Coroners, for whom these investigations were made

REFERENCES

BROUGHTON, P. M. G. (1956), A rapid ultraviolet spectrophotometric method for the detection, estimation and identification of barbiturates in biological material, *Biochem. J.*, **63**, 207–213.

CURRY, A. S. (1963), Rapid method of screening for barbiturates, *Br. med. J.*, **2**, 1040–1041.

—, and SUNSHINE, I. (1960), The liver: blood ratio in cases of barbiturate poisoning, *Toxicol. appl. pharmacol.*, **2**, 602–606.

MOGHRABI, H. M., and CURRY, A. S. (1970), Study of the factors affecting barbiturate levels in post-mortem livers, *Jordan med. J.*, **5**, 10–16.

Post-mortem Morphine and Methadone Levels

ANN E. ROBINSON
Department of Forensic Medicine, The London Hospital Medical College

A few years ago, at the time when there was a growing public concern about the increase in the number of heroin addicts in this country, our curiosity was aroused by the autopsy findings in some sudden deaths from intravenous narcotism reported by Siegel *et al.* (1966). The illicit drugs then available in New York and London were not comparable in that the drug on the London market was in tablet form arising from over-prescription whereas that in New York was in powder form, usually diluted and of variable composition. It appeared worthwhile to investigate addict deaths in London at least for purposes of comparison and also to try to remedy the almost total lack of human toxicological data for drugs of dependence. Why, for example, do some addicts die with a syringe needle still inserted in a vein? Does the answer lie in the manner of injection, the nature of the injected fluid or in the blood level of the drug? Could analysis assist the pathologist in arriving at *the* cause for death as opposed to *a* cause of death? These and many other questions stimulated the work on the dead addicts at The London Hospital Medical College.

It soon became apparent that the lack of published data, both for animals and man, could be attributed to the lack of sufficiently sensitive and specific analytical methods. At the outset, the contemporary problem was that of addiction to heroin and cocaine. Heroin is, of course, rapidly de-acetylated following administration so that the first priority was to establish a suitable quantitative method for the determination of morphine in biological fluids and tissues. The method published in 1971 is still in use (Robinson and Williams, 1971a).

With the passing of time, drug habits changed and quantitative methods for methadone were established and also published (Robinson and Williams, 1971b). Throughout, qualitative tests for drugs have been used to establish the nature of the drugs present prior to quantitative analysis.

The results that have accrued during the past five-and-a-half years now permit tentative interpretation of cases even when the history is incomplete. Some of the results will be discussed under three headings: cases involving morphine, cases involving methadone, and those involving both morphine and methadone. It is not uncommon to find at least one other drug in the autopsy specimens in addition to morphine or methadone but I have selected those in which only minor, in terms of pharmacological significance, amounts of other substances were found.

All of the cases analysed arose from deaths reported to a coroner. Full chemical investigation was carried out on all persons 'known to the Home Office' and also when there was evidence of injection site scarring at autopsy even though the usual enquiries may have failed to elicit any specific indication of drug use. Also, the cases analysed were not limited to those of suspected overdosage.

MORPHINE

Comparatively few of the cases in our records were found to contain morphine only or to contain morphine as the only significant drug at autopsy.

The blood level was not always measurable: levels of 0·33, 0·33, 0·40, and 0·73 μg. morphine per ml. have been found in acute deaths where there was suspicion of so-called 'Chinese Heroin'. In contrast, a 32-year-old male, addicted for about 4 years, found dead in bed had a blood level of 0·039 μg. morphine per ml. Another with a very long history of drug dependence, died some 8 hours after a 30 mg. intravenous dose of heroin, having been given 30 mg. six-hourly for the last few days in a hospital: the blood level at autopsy was less than 0·005 μg. morphine per ml. (*Table* 1).

Table 1. Quantitative results of autopsy specimens from a 46-year-old male who died 8 hours after receiving 30 mg. heroin intravenously and having had 30 mg. heroin intravenously every 6 hours for the previous 4 days.

*Tissue**	*Total morphine (μg. per ml. or g.)*
Peripheral blood	< 0·05
Liver blood	< 0·05
Bile	4·25
Right kidney	1·10
Left kidney	2·20

*Morphine was not detected in any other tissues.

There does not seem to be much future in trying to interpret isolated blood levels of morphine, as is also true of most other drugs, and even consideration of the results for bile and urine in addition is not entirely satisfactory. It may be constructive, however, to consider the proportion of free and bound morphine as well as the absolute levels in the bile and urine. Bound, in this context, refers to morphine present in the conjugated form which may be recovered after preliminary chemical hydrolysis. In the living, some free morphine is excreted in the urine in the period immediately following heroin administration but the proportion of the conjugate increases with time (Williams, 1971). Presumably also the bile will show parallel fluctuations and, because of the entero-hepatic circulation, the bile content may show accumulation as a consequence of previous dosage. A 28-year-old male who had prescribed for him 200 mg. heroin daily in addition to cocaine and methadone and who died following injection of barbiturate had 330 μg. bound morphine and 9·5 μg. free morphine per ml. of bile at autopsy. Conversely, in a death following acute dosage the blood morphine level was not measurable and the bile contained 48·7 μg. total morphine per ml. of which 47·5 μg. per ml. was free morphine.

With regard to tissues, the proportion of bound morphine (protein-bound and conjugate, if present) usually exceeds free morphine in the liver (8 out of 9 cases) and kidney (6 out of 8 cases). The total morphine concentration in the liver exceeds that in the lung (5 out of 5 cases) but other relationships are less well defined, notably the comparison of the liver and kidney levels.

METHADONE

The data for eleven cases have been published (Robinson and Williams, 1971b) and the results for five more recent cases are shown in *Table* 2.

Table 2. Quantitative data for methadone and its cyclic metabolite in autopsy specimens

Tissue and substance	*Case and values (μg. per ml. or g.)* 1* Male 33 years	2 Female 22 years	3 Male 21 years	4 Male 31 years	5 Female 27 years
Blood methadone	2·4	0·98	0·72	1·14	1·25
Blood metabolite	0·35	–	+	0·08	–
Liver blood methadone	2·89	0·08	3·36	0·77	0·49
Liver blood metabolite	–	–	+	0·06	0·12
Bile methadone	20·2	75·0	6·46	10·62	4·00
Bile metabolite	4·52	315·0	20·12	23·17	29·0
Urine methadone	12·02	32·0	3·99	13·87	13·0
Urine metabolite	2·73	58·5	1·14	3·50	0·5
Liver methadone	0·045	6·68	4·85	3·13	2·10
Liver metabolite	0·12	2·7	0·14	0·08	0·08
Right kidney methadone	0·18	5·5	–	1·92	0·18
Right kidney metabolite	0·59	1·33	0·77	+	< 0·04
Left kidney methadone	0·27	3·29	–	1·61	–
Left kidney metabolite	0·47	1·35	–	+	0·04
Spleen methadone	0·045	25·0	2·08	2·99	2·40
Spleen metabolite	0·16	0·95	–	+	+
Right lung methadone	22·25	28·9	4·17	4·32	2·30
Right lung metabolite	0·20	0·53	–	0·12	0·16
Left lung methadone	11·13	23·6	–	5·99	1·80
Left lung metabolite	0·27	0·51	–	+	+
Total methadone in stomach contents (mg.)	200	28·5	–	7·6	60

*Minor amounts of intermediate-acting barbiturate, morphine, and salicylate present.

The brief circumstances were as follows:

Case 1 A 33-year-old male found dead was known to use heroin and methadone.

Case 2 A 22-year-old female who took an oral overdose; a suspension containing 3·5 per cent (w/v) methadone hydrochloride was found whereas 0·18 g. per 100 ml. had been dispensed.

Case 3 A 21-year-old male found dead after 5 days in a warm room.

Case 4 A 31-year-old male who was given 40 mg. methadone at 16.00 hr. and another 40 mg. at 18.00 hr., both orally, who felt dizzy at 21.30 hr., went to bed at 22.30 hr. and was found dead at 07.45 hr. the following day.

Case 5 A 27-year-old male; another case of overdosage in circumstances of reduced tolerance.

The blood levels were all within the range found previously (Robinson and Williams, 1971b), and in two cases the cyclic metabolite was present in sufficient quantity to be measured. Again the blood levels were less than those for other tissues. In the bile specimens, the metabolite concentration exceeded that of methadone, as found previously; likewise in the urine samples, the methadone levels exceeded the metabolite.

In the tissues: the liver concentrations were approximately equal to, or at least of the same order as in the spleen. The lung concentrations exceeded liver, sometimes to a very large factor. Note also that the results for left and right kidneys did not always agree.

The data for these cases are comparable with those previously published and show that the hazard of fatal oral overdosage with methadone still exists.

METHADONE AND MORPHINE

What now of the cases in which both morphine and methadone were found? Interpretation depends upon consideration of the full analytical results and bearing in mind our better documentation for methadone, we usually start with the data for that drug. The only way to present this information is as individual cases.

Case 6 An 18-year-old male was found dead in bed and the room had been cleaned up by his companions. He was thought to have been barbiturate-dependent and a general practitioner had prescribed pentobarbitone sodium (injection), Tuinal, and amphetamine some 3 weeks before his death. A year earlier he had experimented with methadone and 'speed balls' and this had resulted in his having psychiatric treatment. From consideration of the various items found, the deceased had methadone linctus, and injection solution, and phenobarbitone solution for injection available to him, in addition to the prescribed drugs. The quantitative results are shown in *Table* 3. The following points are of interest:

1. Methadone, but not the metabolite, and free morphine were found in the blood.
2. The liver blood level of methadone exceeded that of blood.
3. The lack of the methadone metabolite in the tissues supports the suspicion of an acute fatal dose of methadone, as opposed to chronic dosage. The absolute levels are not easy to interpret because of the problem of assessing tolerance: even if the dosage was accurately known, one does not know what blood or tissue levels to associate with it.

Table 3. Quantitative results of autopsy specimens from Case 6 (Male 18 years)*

Tissue	*Methadone (µg. per ml. or g.)*		*Morphine (µg. per ml. or g.)*			*Amphetamine*
	Per Se	Metabolite	Free	Conjugated	Total	*(µg. per ml. or g.)*
Blood	0·5	–	1·2	–	1·2	7·0
Liver blood	9·4	0·3	0·9	–	0·9	1·1
Bile	23·0	8·2	0·9	0·4	1·3	1·7
Urine	30·0	0·6	3·45	–	3·45	30·4
Liver	1·9	–	0·35	0·5	0·85	0·11
Lung	5·6	–	0·5	0·35	0·85	2·9
Spleen	1·5	–	0·65	–	0·65	0·11
Kidney	0·85	–	0·20	1·05	1·25	0·37
Brain	1·15	–	0·45	1·05	1·5	0·25
Stomach contents (8 ml.)	36·0					

* Morphine was present in injection site tissue from right and left antecubital fossae, left thigh, and left side of neck. Heroin and morphine were detected in tissue from an injection site on the chest.

4. The liver blood level of morphine exceeds that in the peripheral blood, presumably because it (or heroin) was injected.

5. The lack of conjugated morphine in the urine suggested a recent dose of heroin (or morphine) since more free morphine than conjugated is excreted following administration, whereas later proportionately more of the conjugate(s) is present.

6. The presence of bound morphine in the tissues is probably indicative of chronic dosage.

7. The tissue level of total morphine found in the liver and lung are of the same order as expected although more free morphine was present in the lung than in the liver and again this is indicative of recent dosage. This equilibrium is not apparent for methadone. From previous cases, it is expected that the methadone concentrations in the liver and lung are approximately equivalent when methadone is the only drug involved and when the survival time between dose and death is 8 to 9 hours. This again supports the contention of a comparatively short survival time after the last dose.

8. Amphetamine was present in the specimens and the distribution of it is shown in *Table* 3. The cause of death given by the pathologist was heroin and methadone poisoning.

Case 7 The deceased was a 20-year-old male, who was found collapsed in a house and was dead on arrival at hospital. He was a known addict with a four or five year history of drug use and many old injection sites on both arms. Qualitative analysis of autopsy specimens revealed the presence of morphine, methadone, and intermediate-acting barbiturate. Tissue from an injection site showed only the barbiturate. Swabs from the hands showed positive evidence for the presence of cannabis constituents. The quantitative results are shown in *Table* 4. The following points are of interest:

1. Although a barbiturate was found in a syringe needle and in an injection site, there was no measurable blood level (< 0·1 mg. per 100 ml.). The amount in the urine may be indicative of administration some time before death. However, it is conceivable that collapse occurred during or immediately after injection.

2. Methadone was not detectable in the blood (limit 0·5 μg. in 10 ml. sample).

Table 4. Quantitative analysis of autopsy specimens from Case 7 (Male 20 years)

Tissue	*Methadone*★ (*μg. per ml. or g.*)	*Morphine (μg. per ml. or g.)* Free	Conjugated	Total
Blood†	–	0·97	–	0·97
Bile	33·5	8·9	0·1	59·0
Urine‡	23·5	0·4	25·8	26·2
Liver	0·9	1·9	–	1·9
Lung	3·45	1·35	0·8	2·55
Spleen	0·1	1·5	0·83	2·33
Kidney	0·9	1·05	2·3	3·35
Brain	–	1·35	2·85	4·2
Stomach contents (450 g.)	4·5	ca. 30·0		

★Metabolite not detected in any specimen.
†Barbiturate not detected.
‡Intermediate-acting barbiturate present 1·1 mg. per 100 ml., calculated as amylobarbitone.

3. The presence of methadone in the stomach may be the remains of an oral dose or may be the consequence of secretion of the drug in the gastric juice. Gastric secretion of methadone has been apparent in previous cases when there was no oral dose form of the drug available. Nicotine is likewise found in the gastric content of smokers.

4. The methadone levels of the liver and kidney are equivalent but the drug level is higher in relation to liver than is usual and, but for the 'negative' blood level, would imply recent dosage.

5. Morphine was present free in the blood and also in the gastric content.

6. Tissue levels of morphine in liver, lung, and kidney are again not equivalent but the excess morphine over the conjugated or bound form is consistent with recent dosage.

The cause of death given by the pathologist was 'morphine and methadone poisoning'. The coroner's verdict was 'drug addiction'.

Case 8 This was the case of a 22-year-old garage mechanic with a four-year history of drug use. Nine months before his death he had been receiving methadone linctus on prescription. He went abroad, returning to this country some four weeks before he died. On the night of his death he locked the door of his room while his girl friend went to have a bath. Unable to enter the room she called the landlord who used the passkey. By then he was unconscious on the floor, and was dead on arrival at hospital. A used syringe, but no needle, and a small box containing screwed-up paper were the only items found by the Coroner's Officer. The deceased was alleged to have bought 'Chinese heroin', and the powder residue on the paper did indeed contain heroin, 6-monoacetyl morphine, morphine, caffeine, and

Table 5. Quantitative results of autopsy specimens from Case 8 (Male 22 years)

Tissue	*Morphine (μg. per ml. or g.)* Total	Free	*Methadone (μg. per ml. or g.)* Per Se	Metabolite
Blood	–	–	–	–
Bile	50·8	4·2	–	–
Urine	20·2	5·45	0·63	+
Liver	0·75	+	0·45	–
Right lung	1·25	+	1·03	–
Left lung	1·05	0·85	0·98	–
Spleen	0·85	+	0·09	–
Right kidney	1·75	0·65	–	–
Left kidney	1·75	0·95	–	–
Brain	+	+	–	–
Stomach contents (total)	–	–	–	–

acetylated codeine. The results for the fluid specimens (*Table* 5) showed no detectable morphine or methadone in the blood, and most conjugated morphine in the bile and urine. Tissues showed, however, that of the morphine present most of it was free, consistent with recent dosage (*Table* 5). Neither of the suspected injection sites yielded morphine or methadone. It was concluded that the last drug administered had been heroin, and the pathologist gave morphine and methadone poisoning as the cause of death.

A further case was presented in which the inconsistency of the analytical results gave rise to suspicion of malfunction of the liver, which was confirmed by the histological findings (Robinson and Holder, 1973).

There are three conclusions that may be drawn from this work:

1. One cannot reasonably interpret isolated results.
2. Chemical diagnosis of a pathological condition is possible.
3. One can never rely on 'hearsay' evidence of drug use, and that care is appropriate even with prescribing records.

Acknowledgements: I am indebted to H.M. Coroners and my pathologist colleagues for their help and co-operation, and to Miss Waller for her technical assistance.

REFERENCES

ROBINSON, A. E., and HOLDER, A. T. (1973), Contemporary trends in drug abuse in London as reflected by toxicological investigations of autopsy specimens. *Z. Rechtsmedizin.*, **72**, 306–311.

—, and WILLIAMS, F. M. (1971a), Post-mortem distribution of morphine in heroin addicts, *Medicine Sci. Law*, **11**, 135–138.

— — (1971b), The distribution of methadone in man, *J. Pharm. Pharmac.*, **23**, 353–358.

SIEGEL, H., HELPERN, M., and EHRENREICH, T. (1966), The diagnosis of death from intravenous narcotism. With emphasis on the pathologic aspects, *J. forens. Sci.*, **11**, 1–16.

WILLIAMS, F. M. (1971), Ph.D. Thesis, University of London.

Hallucinogens

R. W. BRIMBLECOMBE
Medical Division, Chemical Defence Establishment, Porton Down *

The purpose of this paper is to define, classify, and indicate something of what is known of the mode of action of hallucinogenic drugs. A good many of the drugs to be mentioned have been, and still are, abused, some in specific areas of the world, others more or less universally. For this reason they are of interest to the forensic scientist. No attempt will be made here, however, to describe methods for their detection; these are to be found in textbooks of forensic toxicology or in recent research papers.

The term hallucinogen is not a particularly apt one for the drugs which will be discussed, since hallucinations do not necessarily form a regular part of the syndrome produced by all of them. It is difficult, however, to find a satisfactory alternative. Psychotomimetic is a commonly used term but the implication of this word, that the effects of the drugs mimic those observed in naturally-occurring psychoses, is no longer acceptable for the great majority of the drugs. A W.H.O. Study Group on Psychotropic Drugs which met in 1966 suggested the term psychodysleptic but this has not passed into common usage. Given this difficulty in nomenclature it is necessary to have a precise definition of the drugs to be discussed. That produced by Downing in 1962 (to describe 'psychotomimetic drugs') will be used here. It reads 'a drug which will consistently produce changes in thought, perception and mood, occurring alone or in concert, without causing major disturbances of the autonomic nervous system or other serious disability'.

This definition stresses the specificity and reproducibility of the effects of the drugs and excludes a very wide range of chemical substances which have been reported as producing aberrant behaviour, but only occasionally, and then often in hypersensitive individuals, or after gross overdosage, and even then usually accompanied by other, non-behavioural, effects.

Since there is still considerable ignorance concerning the modes and sites of action of hallucinogenic drugs there is some difficulty in classifying them in a logical and reliable manner. At the present state of knowledge the best classification is:

1. Sympathomimetic amines
   a. Indoleamines
   b. Phenylalkylamines
2. Anticholinergics
3. Cannabis
4. Miscellaneous

*Present address: The Research Institute, Smith, Kline and French Laboratories, Welwyn Garden City, Herts.

It is virtually certain, as will be discussed later, that the modes of action of the drugs in these various groups are quite different despite the fact that they produce effects which are superficially similar. There is also the possibility that drugs within these groups, especially the first one, do not share a common mode of action. Further evidence is required before this question can be resolved. The miscellaneous compounds represent such a heterogeneous group that they will not be dealt with here.

SYMPATHOMIMETIC AMINES

Indoleamines

It has been stated (Robinson, 1968) that about a quarter of all known alkaloids are indole-containing compounds. Many of these are hallucinogens and form the active principles of various preparations used for centuries in different parts of the world, but notably by the Mexican Indians, to produce hallucinations and other behavioural effects in religious rituals.

The simplest hallucinogenic idoleamines are *N,N*-dialkyltryptamines (I)

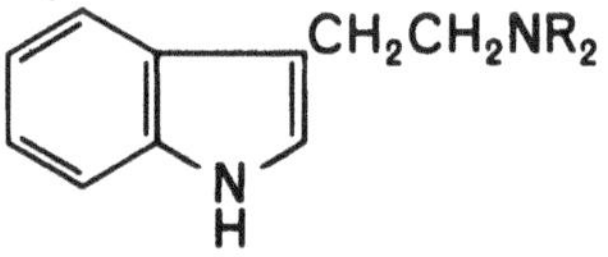

(I)

These include *N,N*-dimethyltryptamine (I, R=CH_3), which produces short-lived behavioural effects in man after intramuscular doses of about 1 mg. per kg. (Szara, 1956), and the closely related *N,N*-diethyltryptamine (I, R=C_2H_5) and *N,N*-dipropyltryptamine (I, R=nC_3H_7) which are effective at about the same dose levels through the effects are longer-lasting than those of the dimethyl compound (Szara and Hearst, 1962). Despite the close chemical resemblance between these compounds there appear to be qualitative differences in the syndromes produced. For example Boszormenyi, Der, and Nagy (1959) reported that *N,N*-diethyltryptamine led to a pleasant, meditative, euphoric state in contrast to *N,N*-dimethyltryptamine which caused anxiety and disturbances of mood and perception. *N,N*-dibutyltryptamine (I, R=C_4H_9) is less active than the lower homologues and the *N,N*-dihexyl compound (I, R=hexyl) completely lacks activity (Szara, 1961). The evidence suggests (Szara, 1956; Shulgin, 1970) that the active compounds in this series are effective only when administered parenterally, not when given by mouth.

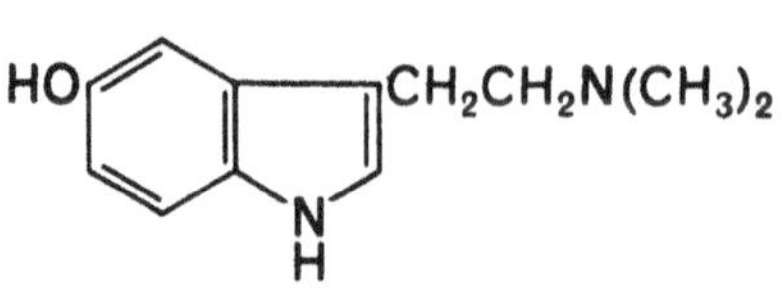

(II)

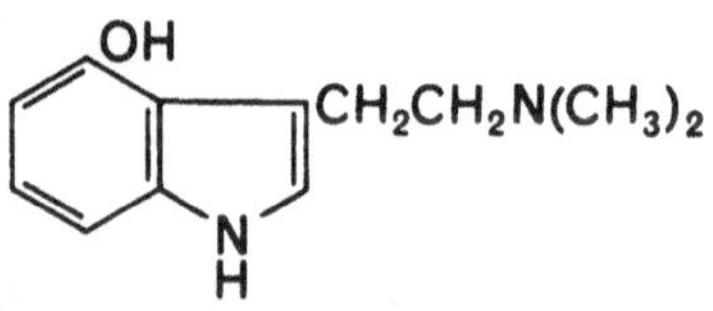

(III)

Other well-known hallucinogenic tryptamine derivatives with substituents in the benzene ring as well as on the side-chain nitrogen atom are bufotenine (5-hydroxy-*N,N*-dimethyltryptamine, II) and psilocin (4-hydroxy-*N,N*-dimethyltrypt-amine, III).

Fabing and Hawkins (1956) reported that intravenous doses of from 2 to 16 mg. per kg. bufotenine caused behavioural changes but Isbell (1967) found the compound to be inactive when given by mouth or by inhalation. There is no doubt about the activity of psilocin when given by mouth. In an early paper Hofmann *et al.* (1958) reported that oral doses of from 4 to 8 mg. per man (approximately 60–120 μg per kg.) were effective in producing effects similar to those produced by mescaline or lysergic acid diethylamide (LSD-25). Hollister (1961) confirmed that 60 μg. per kg. by mouth was the threshold dose and in a comparative study Wolbach, Miner, and Isbell (1962) confirmed the similarities in the syndromes produced by psilocin, mescaline and LSD-25.

A few other tryptamine derivatives have been tested in man but there is insufficient quantitative information to enable meaningful conclusions to be drawn concerning the precise relationship between structure and hallucinogenic activity. There have, however, been some animal studies from which some conclusions can be drawn if it is assumed that the behavioural effects studied are relevant to hallucinogenic activity. For example, Gessner *et al.* (1968) studied compounds with methoxy substitution at positions 4,5,6, and 7 in the benzene ring and with alkyl substituents on the side-chain nitrogen atom. They used blockade of a conditioned avoidance response of rats in a shuttle-box as their criterion of activity. Methoxy substitution at positions 4 or 5 conferred greater activity than corresponding substitution at positions 6 or 7. Dimethyl or diethyl substituents on the side-chain nitrogen atom gave equal activity.

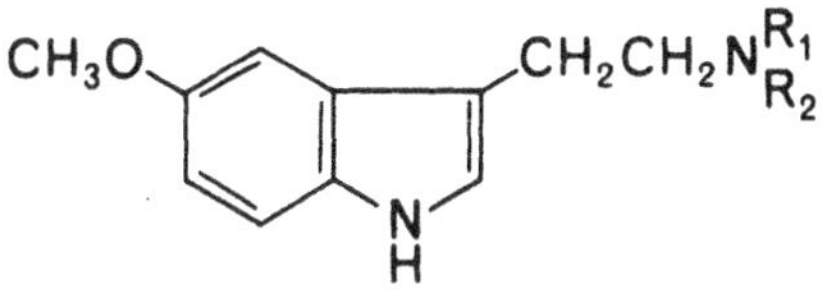

(IV)

Three of the compounds studied, *N,N*-dimethyl-5-methoxytryptamine (IV, $R_1 = R_2 = CH_3$), *N,N*-diethyl-5-methoxtryptamine (IV, $R_1 = R_2 = C_2H_5$) and *N,N*-methylethyl-5-methoxytryptamine (IV, $R_1 = CH_3$, $R_2 = C_2H_5$) were more active in this test than either psilocin or *N,N*-diethyl-tryptamine.

In another study Brimblecombe (1967) showed a good correlation between the potencies of 36 tryptamine derivatives in modifying rat behaviour in an open-field test situation and in causing hyperthermia in rabbits; the latter response seems to give a good indication of hallucinogenic activity. Some general conclusions concerning structure-activity relationships were drawn. Substitution with lower alkyl groups on the side-chain nitrogen conferred higher activity than higher alkyl substitution. Among the active compounds dialkyl substitution produced more active compounds than corresponding mono-alkyl substitution. In the few cases where comparisons were possible substitution in the benzene ring always reduced activity. These general rules did not hold where the side-chain nitrogen was incorporated into a pyrrolidine ring. This tended to increase the lethal toxicity; the most active and the most lethal of the compounds studied was *N,N*-tetramethylene-5-methoxytryptamine (V)

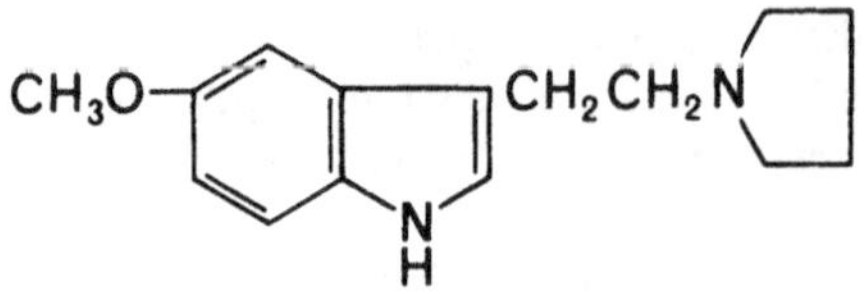

(V)

Without doubt the most active indoleamine hallucinogen is LSD-25 (VI, $R^1 = N(C_2H_5)_2$, $R^2 = R^3 = H$)

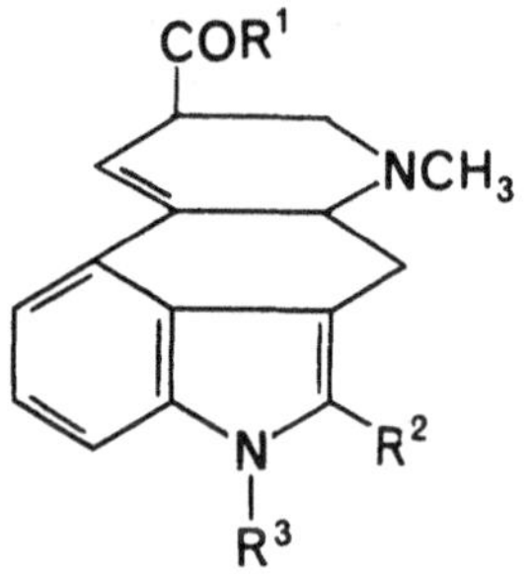

(VI)

This is active in man in doses of about 0·5–1 μg. per kg. and appears to be equally effective whether given by mouth or by parenteral injection. Even small changes in the structure result in dramatic decreases in activity. In a study reported in 1960 Hofmann compared the hallucinogenic activities in man of 18 derivatives of lysergic acid with their hyperthermic activities in rabbits and their *in vitro* activities in antagonizing the effects of 5-hydroxytryptamine (VII; serotonin; 5-HT).

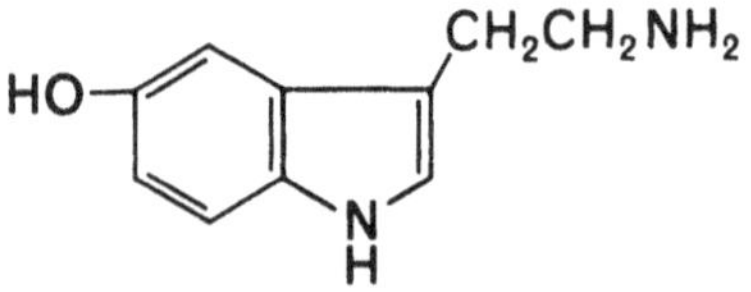

(VII)

Hallucinogenic activity was reduced when the diethylamino group of LSD-25 at R^1 was replaced by other amines but some activity still remained. When the double bond in the D ring was saturated there was almost complete loss of activity as there was with substitution at R^2 (e.g. 2-bromo-LSD; BOL-148; VI, R^3 = Br). However, certain substituents at R^3 (e.g. 1-acetyl-LSD; VI, R^3 = acetyl) gave compounds almost as active as LSD-25.

Phenylalkylamines

Many phenylalkylamines are found in nature and, like the indoleamines, some of them are responsible for the effects of concoctions used in religious rites and ceremonies. A typical compound is mescaline (VIII, 3,4,5-trimethoxyphenylethylamine) which is found in various species of cactus, particularly *Lophophora williamsii* (the peyotl cactus).

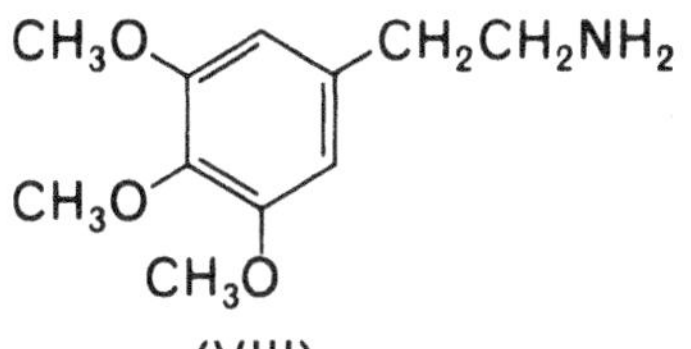

(VIII)

Mescaline is not very potent in comparison with LSD-25 or even some of the simple tryptamines. The average effective oral dose in man is about 0·3–0·6 g. (i.e. 4–8 mg. per kg.). Most workers agree that the effects are very similar to those produced by LSD-25.

There have been a number of studies of the activity of structural analogues of mescaline. For example, De Jong (1945) investigated a number of phenylethylamine derivatives for their 'catatonizing action' and 'fear-producing activity' in cats. Whether either of these effects can be related to hallucinogenic activity is doubtful but none of the compounds studied was significantly more potent than mescaline itself, although 3,4-dimethyoxyphenylethylamine (IX, DMPEA) had approximately equal activity.

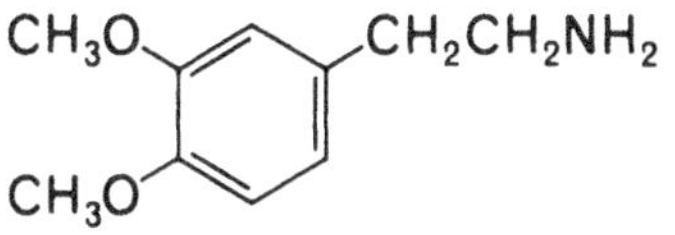

(IX)

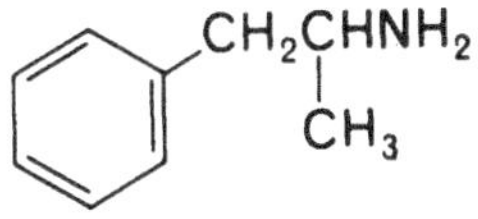

(X)

The latter compound aroused considerable interest a few years ago as 'pink-spot' when it was claimed to be present in the urine of schizophrenics but not in that of non-schizophrenic subjects (Friedhoff and Van Winkel, 1962). Other workers have since refuted this claim (e.g. Perry *et al.*, 1966), and, in any case, Shulgin, Sargent, and Naranjo (1966) could detect no behavioural or autonomic disturbances when the compound was administered to man.

Compounds with considerably enhanced hallucinogenic potency result from α-methyl substitution, i.e. to give derivatives of amphetamine (X).

Amphetamine itself does not conform to the definition of an hallucinogenic drug used here although there is now ample evidence for the occurrence of a schizophrenia-like psychosis in chronic users of the drug. Many substituted amphetamines, however, are hallucinogens. One of the earliest to be investigated was 3,4,5-trimethoxyphenylisopropylamine (XI, $R^2 = R^3 = R^4 = OCH_3$, $R^1 = H$; TMA) which was shown to be about twice as active as mescaline in man (Peretz,

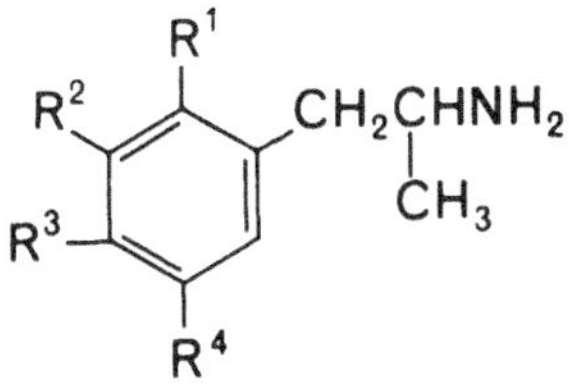

(XI)

Smythies, and Gibson, 1955). Since then numerous substituted amphetamines have been investigated by Shulgin and his colleagues (Shulgin, Sargent, and Naranjo, 1969; Shulgin, 1970) and their structure-activity relationships analysed. One important structural feature, already referred to, is the length of the side chain with the 3 carbon atom side chain of the amphetamine conferring higher activity than the unbranched 2 carbon atom chain of the phenylethylamines. Increase in the chain length to 4 leads to a decrease in activity. The effects of methoxyl substitution in the *ortho, meta,* and *para* positions in the ring were also analysed. *Ortho* substitution (i.e. at R^1, in XI) led to an increase in activity while *meta* substitution (at R^2) led to a decrease. The effects of *para* substitution (at R^3) were not so clear. The possibility, suggested by Shulgin and co-workers, that these compounds might be metabolized to indoles which would be responsible for their hallucinogenic activity, is given some support by these findings, since indoles would be more easily formed from *ortho-*, as opposed to *meta-*, substituted compounds.

An interesting compound in Shulgin's series is 2,5-dimethoxy-3,4-methylenedioxamphetamine (XII), which was synthesized because of its resemblance to myristicin (XIII), one of the main constitutents of nutmeg and possibly the substance responsible for the hallucinogenic effects of large doses of nutmeg. This amphetamine derivative was about twelve times as active as mescaline. The most active member of

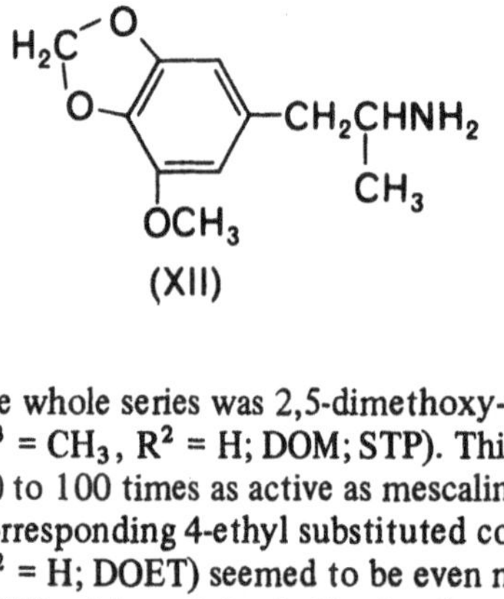

(XII)

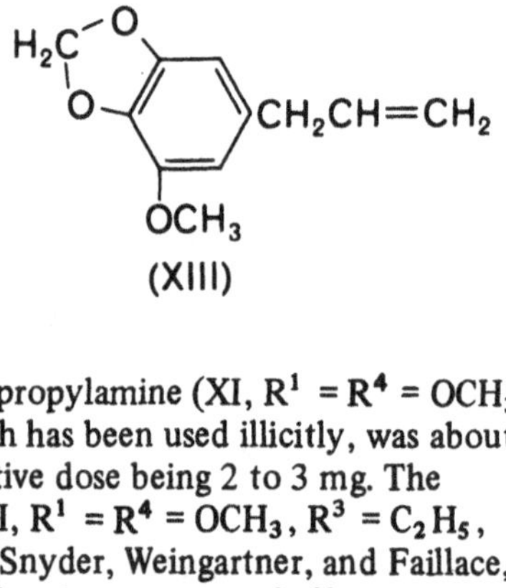

(XIII)

the whole series was 2,5-dimethoxy-4-methylisopropylamine (XI, $R^1 = R^4 = OCH_3$, $R^3 = CH_3$, R^2 = H; DOM; STP). This drug, which has been used illicitly, was about 80 to 100 times as active as mescaline, the effective dose being 2 to 3 mg. The corresponding 4-ethyl substituted compound (XI, $R^1 = R^4 = OCH_3$, $R^3 = C_2H_5$, R^2 = H; DOET) seemed to be even more active (Snyder, Weingartner, and Faillace, 1970) with a minimal effective dose of 1·5 mg., but its spectrum of effects was rather different, with euphoria being predominant at low doses.

There are still a number of possible structural variations to the basic amphetamine molecule and the possibility of the discovery of even more active compounds should not be discounted.

Mode of Action of Sympathomimetic Hallucinogens

Before embarking on a discussion of possible modes of action of the drugs described above it is desirable to list the evidence which seems to justify grouping them altogether into a single category. Five types of evidence exist:

1. Production of similar effects.
2. Similarity in chemical structures.
3. Production of cross-tolerance.
4. Similarity in pharmacological actions.
5. Similarity in biochemical effects.

The first point, the production of similar effects, has already been referred to several times. Various authors have pointed out marked similarities in the syndrome produced by LSD-25, mescaline, psilocin, STP, and various other drugs mentioned above. Since many of the effects produced by the drugs are subjective in nature and hence difficult to specify accurately or to quantify, this type of evidence may not be very strong but is, nevertheless, suggestive of similar modes of action.

Structural resemblances between the tryptamines and LSD-25, which all share the indole nucleus, are obvious, but it is also possible to take the view that the substituted amphetamines have stereochemical and electronic similarities to the hallucinogenic indoleamines and this might interact with a common receptor. This matter has been discussed by a number of authors (Chothia and Pauling, 1969; Snyder and Richelson, 1970; Inch, 1972).

Tolerance develops rapidly to the effects of LSD-25 and cross-tolerance occurs between this drug and psilocybin (Hollister, 1961), mescaline (Balestrieri, 1957), and STP (Green, 1972). There is no cross-tolerance between LSD-25 and D-amphetamine (Rosenberg *et al.*, 1963) but this might be expected on the grounds that the latter drug is not an hallucinogen. Less easy to explain is the lack of cross-tolerance between LSD-25 and *N,N*-dimethyltryptamine (Rosenberg *et al.*, 1964) but in general the existence of this cross-tolerance is indicative of common modes of action or at least of common final pathways in the modes of action.

Similarities in the pharmacological actions of the compounds in this group will become apparent later in this section where detailed modes of action are discussed. It is sufficient at this stage to note again that the drugs are all sympathomimetics, i.e. they all produce effects identical to those resulting from stimulation of the sympathetic nervous system. These include increase in blood pressure and in heart rate, piloerection and hyperglycaemia. However, it is not true to say that all sympathomimetic drugs are hallucinogens. An example is amphetamine which, as has already been noted, is not an hallucinogen. The reasons for this are not understood. It may simply be a matter of access to different brain areas or there may be more fundamental differences, such as interaction with different receptors.

Some of the biochemical actions of the sympathomimetic hallucinogens are described below and again there is evidence for similar actions of drugs within the group.

Taken together, the evidence summarized thus far seems to be strongly indicative of similar, if not identical, modes of action.

Pharmacology and Biochemistry of Sympathomimetic Hallucinogens

Neuropharmacological studies with hallucinogens have, in the main, concentrated on their effects on synaptic transmission in specific systems, on the spontaneous electrical activity of the cortex and on evoked potentials.

The effects of LSD-25 on synaptic transmission have been studied widely. The early work was summarized by Evarts (1957) but the overall picture is a confused one. Purpura (1956), for example, studied the effects of the drug on evoked potentials in the auditory and visual systems and concluded that axodendritic transmission was inhibited while axosomatic transmission was facilitated; indeed, it is apparent from the work of a number of authors that synapses differ markedly in their sensitivity to LSD-25, although the effect most commonly reported is inhibition, especially in the lateral geniculate nucleus in the visual pathway. Similar effects have also been reported for the hallucinogens bufotenine, psilocybin, *N,N*-dimethyltryptamine, and mescaline (Marrazzi and Hart, 1953; Evarts, 1958;

Bishop *et al.*, 1960; Marrazzi, 1960) but also for the non-hallucinogenic substances tryptamine and BOL-148. Curtis and Davis (1962) studied the effects of a number of compounds ejected electrophoretically frcm multi-barrelled micro-pipettes on the excitation of lateral geniculate neurones by volleys in optic nerve fibres. The putative neurotransmitter substance 5-hydroxtryptamine (VII, serotonin, 5-HT) depressed the excitation either, it was suggested, by interfering with the synthesis or preventing the release of the excitatory transmitter or by preventing its interaction with post-synaptic receptor sites. A number of compounds structurally related to 5-HT had similar depressant actions. These compounds included hydroxytryptamines, *N*-alkyltryptamines, and lysergic acid derivatives, many of proven hallucinogenic activity and it was suggested that depressant actions on synaptic transmission elsewhere in the central nervous system might account for this activity.

The clearest effects of LSD-25 on the spontaneous electrical activity of the brain is to cause a decrease in amplitude of the electro-encephalogram (E.E.G.). Bradley and Elkes (1953, 1957) studied the effects of LSD-25 on various cat preparations and showed that in the conscious unrestrained animal the E.E.G. pattern was very similar to that seen in the normal alert animal. This pattern was not produced by the drug in *encéphale isolé* preparations with the spinal cord sectioned at C1, implying that spinal connections were necessary for the 'alerting' effect of LSD-25. In fact it was postulated that its action was to facilitate input into the brain stem reticular formation. In contrast certain hallucinogenic tryptamine derivatives studied by Bradley and Marley (1965) seemed not to require the presence of sensory input to produce E.E.G. alerting in cats.

Rinaldi and Himwich (1955) found that the effects of mescaline on the E.E.G. were almost identical with those of LSD-25.

The effects of LSD-25 on evoked potentials in cats have been studied, among others, by Key (1965a,b) and, more recently, by Green and Aldous (1972). The amplitudes of evoked potentials (EPs) in a specific sensory pathway, the lateral lemniscus (LL), are reasonably steady under sound-proofed conditions whereas under distractive conditions they are reduced but more variable. LSD-25 produces an effect similar to that produced by distractive conditions. It seems (Galambos, 1960) that the degree of fluctuation in amplitude of EPs may be related to the significance attached to the stimulus so that LSD-25 seems to increase the significance of stimuli. Effects on cortical evoked potentials are more complex but lead to essentially the same conclusion. Very little similar work seems to have been carried out with other sympathomimetic hallucinogens.

The general conclusion to be drawn from neuropharmacological studies with LSD-25 is that the drug modifies in various ways the passage of sensory impulses through the brain. The result of this is, presumably, that the sensory information is misinterpreted in the sensory cortex leading to the distortions in perception characteristic of the drug. The limited evidence which is available suggests that other sympathomimetic hallucinogens have essentially the same actions although there are certain detailed differences which cannot, at present, be explained.

Biochemically, there have been numerous studies with LSD-25. In the main there seems to be little consistency in the results which vary with dose of drug, species of animal used, etc. However, the actions of LSD-25 and of other sympathomimetic hallucinogens upon levels of brain amines seem to produce a consistent pattern which warrants serious consideration.

The interactions of LSD-25 with putative transmitter substances in the brain have been of interest since Gaddum (1953) showed that it antagonised the action of 5-HT on the isolated rat uterus. This led naturally to the suggestion that this antagonistic action of the drug at central serotoninergic synapses was responsible for its hallucinogenic actions. However, it was soon discovered (Cerletti and Rothlin, 1955) that the non-hallucinogenic BOL-148 was also a potent antagonist of 5-HT on isolated smooth muscle and it was concluded from this and other evidence that antagonism of 5-HT was of no relevance in the central actions of LSD-25 (Costa *et al.*, 1962). This conclusion may need careful re-examination in the light of a recent report by Boakes *et al.* (1970) that in experiments where drugs were applied to brain stem neurones by microiontophoresis the excitatory actions of 5-HT were antagonized by LSD-25 but not by BOL-148.

There is now ample proof that LSD-25 causes elevation in levels of 5-HT in the brain with concomitant reductions in the concentrations of noradrenaline (Freedman, 1961). This has led to the suggestion (Freedman and Aghajanian, 1966) that shifts in the equilibrium of amines at central sites are of importance in the mode of action of the drug. More recently the effects of hallucinogenic drugs have been analysed in detail by Tonge and Leonard (1969). They found that in rats doses of LSD-25 and mescaline sufficient to cause behavioural changes gave increases in levels of 5-HT and decreases in levels of its metabolite 5-hydroxyindole acetic acid (5-HIAA). The maximal rise in 5-HT levels corresponded to the peak of the behavioural effects. Increased levels of the amine could result from an increase in its rate of synthesis or a decrease in its rate of metabolic destruction:

$$\text{5-hydroxytryptophan} \xrightarrow[\text{decarboxylase}]{\text{Amino acid}} \text{5-hydroxytryptamine} \xrightarrow[\text{oxidase}]{\text{Monoamine}} \text{5-hydroxyindole acetic acid}$$

(5 HTP) (5 HT) (5 HIAA)

It was found, however, that the drugs produced no alterations in the activity of amino acid decarboxylase or monoamine oxidase, the enzymes responsible for the synthesis and breakdown of 5-HT.

Another possibility is that the hallucinogens affect the rate of release of 5-HT. The drug *p*-chlorophenylalamine causes a depletion of 5-HT by inhibiting the enzyme tryptophan hydroxylase. The hallucinogenic drugs reduced the degree of depletion produced by *p*-chlorophenylalamine suggesting that they decreased the turnover rate of 5-HT. Precisely how this is brought about is not clear but one possibility is that LSD-25 and mescaline interact with 5-HT receptors, an action which has been suggested from time to time, thus decreasing the turnover rate by a feedback mechanism.

In another study Leonard and Tonge (1969) found that LSD-25 and mescaline decreased levels of noradrenaline in rat brain with concomitant slight increase in dopamine. The drug α-methyl-*p*-tyrosine causes depletion of noradrenaline by inhibition of the rate-limiting enzyme tyrosine hydroxylase but the hallucinogenic drugs did not influence the degree of depletion produced. They did, however, increase the depletion of noradrenaline brought about by α-methyl-*m*-tyrosine which acts by replacing noradrenaline in the neuronal storage granules with metaraminol. From this evidence it seemed possible that the hallucinogens inhibited the rate of release of noradrenaline from the neurone, thus allowing its intraneuronal catabolism by monoamine oxidase.

The implication of these biochemical studies seems to be that normal transmitter-receptor interactions at both tryptaminergic and adrenergic sites within the brain are disrupted by the hallucinogenic drugs.

A very important finding by Leonard was that the effects reported above were produced not only by the sympathomimetic hallucinogens LSD-25 and mescaline but also by the non-sympathomimetic drugs Ditran and phencyclidine (see below). This immediately throws doubt on the view expressed earlier in this paper that hallucinogenic drugs in different classes produce their effects via different modes of action. It should be pointed out, however, that the doses of all the drugs used in these experiments (LSD-25 200 μg. per kg., mescaline 10 mg. per kg., Ditran 4 mg. per kg., and phencyclidine 10 mg. per kg.) were very high in relation to the hallucinogenic doses in man and that the effects may represent some relatively non-specific response. The rat appears to be resistant to the effect of these drugs, however, and the doses may be realistic for this species. It is possible that the observed effects on amine levels represent a final common consequence arrived at from different modes of action.

ANTICHOLINERGICS

Anticholinergic drugs, also known as antiacetylcholine drugs, cholinolytics, or atropine-like drugs, have been recognized as hallucinogens ever since it was realized that the belladonna alkaloids, such as atropine (XIV) and hyoscine (XV), were responsible for the signs and symptoms of poisoning by certain solanaceous plants. These signs and symptoms include behavioural disturbances such as hallucinations, mood changes, and depersonalization.

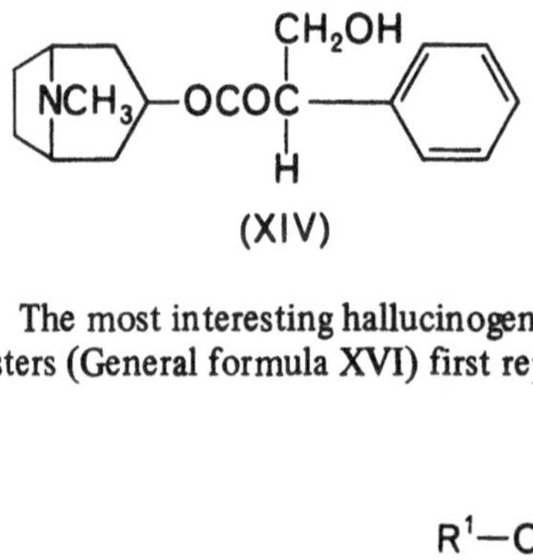

(XIV)

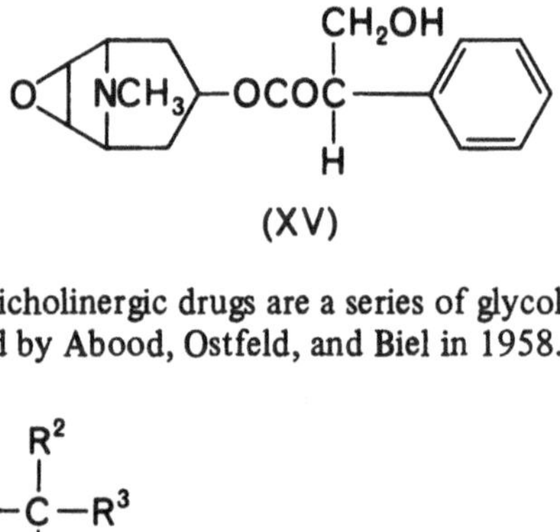

(XV)

The most interesting hallucinogenic anticholinergic drugs are a series of glycollate esters (General formula XVI) first reported by Abood, Ostfeld, and Biel in 1958.

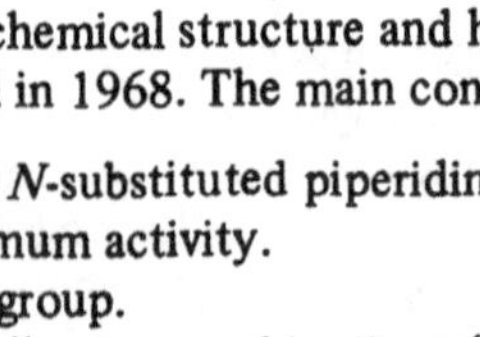

(XVI)

The relationship between chemical structure and hallucinogenic activity of these drugs was reviewed by Abood in 1968. The main conclusions were:

a. In the series where R^1 = *N*-substituted piperidine or pyrolidine, the *N*-substituted must be lower alkyl for maximum activity.

b. R^2 must be a hydroxyl group.

c. R^3 and R^4 can be the following combinations (in decreasing order of activity), cycloalkyl + phenyl; phenyl + phenyl; phenyl + unsaturated alkyl; cycloalkyl + unsaturated alkyl; phenyl + alkyl; cycloalkyl + alkyl; alkyl + alkyl.

d. Activity is lost following substitution of halides, alkyl, alkoxy, or phenyl in one or both phenyl rings of the acid moiety.

e. In the series where R^1 is *N*-substituted piperidine, greatest potency is found with the ester in the 4-position of the ring. The 3-position is less potent and the 2-position least potent of all.

f. The thiol esters where –S– is substituted for –O– are less active and shorter acting.

g. Esters of 3-quinuclidinol compare in activity to the 4-piperidyl-cyclopentyl esters whereas esters of 3-tropanol and 3-granatonol are somewhat less active.

One of the most active and most studied compounds in this series is Ditran (XVII)

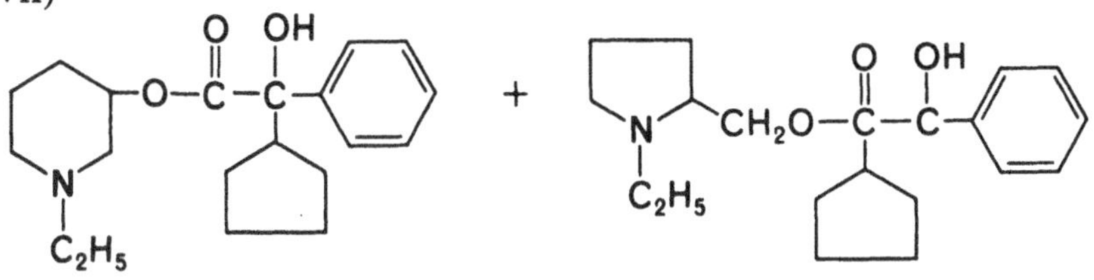

30% 70%

(XVII)

A number of workers have studied the effects of this drug given in doses of between 1 and 25 mg. by mouth or by intramuscular or intravenous injection. Their results have been summarized by Abood (1968), who notes that among the most striking actions of the drug are the hallucinations, which are predominantly visual though other sensory systems may be involved. Amnesia is also a characteristic effect. It has been claimed (for example by Gershon and Olariu, 1960; Finkelstein, 1961) that the syndrome produced by Ditran closely resembles schizophrenia. The fact that most of the reported effects are somewhat unpleasant probably accounts for the fact that drugs of this type have not, to the knowledge of the author, been used illicitly in recent years in Western civilizations. Various preparations of the solanaceous plant *Datura* have been employed for centuries by South American Indian tribes (Brown, 1971). A violent initial reaction is followed by a deep sleep with hallucinations and during this latter period the recipient of the drug is believed to acquire divine powers from visits by the spirits. Other special uses of the drug, also quoted by Brown, include its administration to unmanageable children and to wives who were about to be buried alive with their deceased husbands.

Mode of Action of Anticholinergic Hallucinogens

Peripherally, anticholinergic drugs act as competitive antagonists to acetylcholine at its muscarinic sites of action, i.e. at postganglionic parasympathetic receptors. It is reasonable, therefore, to examine the postulate that the hallucinogenic properties of these drugs are due to similar actions at central acetylcholine receptors. There now seems ample evidence (Bebbington and Brimblecombe, 1965; Brimblecombe, 1970) for the presence of central receptors bearing a close resemblance to peripheral muscarinic receptors. There is, however, still no complete acceptance of the view that anticholinergic drugs produce their hallucinogenic effects by interaction with these receptors.

Some studies (Abood, Ostfeld and Biel, 1959; Lipman, 1967) have failed to show correlations between anticholinergic potency and psychotomimetic or hallucinogenic activity but the tests used for anticholinergic potency were carried out on such preparations as the isolated guinea pig ileum, i.e. they were measures of peripheral, rather than central, activity and thus of little relevance.

Other workers have studied the effects of anticholinergic drugs on the electrical activity of the brain; as a result of such studies Herz (1963) concluded that a common cholinergic mechanism was involved in the effects of a series of such drugs on behaviour and on the electrical activity of the brain. White and Carlton (1963) investigated the effects of some piperidyl glycollates on the E.E.G. of rabbits and suggested that their results supported the hypothesis that these hallucinogens acted via a central anticholinergic mechanism.

A characteristic effect of anticholinergic drugs is to produce a so-called dissociation between E.E.G. and behaviour, i.e. animals under the influence of these drugs can be behaviourally alert while exhibiting E.E.G. patterns normally associated with sleep. Brimblecombe and Green (1967, 1968) were able to show a statistically significant correlation between the central anticholinergic potencies of a series of drugs and their ability to produce this dissociation in cats. This indicates the presence of cholinergic synapses in the neural system involved in E.E.G. arousal but does not necessarily mean that the hallucinogenic action of the drugs results from a blocking action at acetylcholine receptors since the behavioural significance of the dissociation phenomenon is not clear.

Attempts to correlate potency in producing specific behavioural effects with central anticholinergic potency have proved difficult mainly because the drugs induce a state of hyperactivity in experimental animals. This tends to complicate the interpretation of results in, for example, avoidance conditioning situations where the response involves activity of some sort (Brimblecombe and Buxton, 1972).

The real requirement is for more quantitative data on the effects of these drugs on man to enable a statistical comparison to be made between their hallucinogenic potency and their anticholinergic activity.

Although competitive antagonism of acetylcholine still seems the most likely mode of action of these drugs there are other pieces of evidence, not necessarily conflicting, which should be mentioned.

An early finding (Abood and Rinaldi, 1959) was that tritium-labelled *N*-ethyl-3-piperidyl benzilate was localized in the central nervous system predominantly in a cytoplasmic granular fraction which consisted largely of mitochondria and it was concluded that the drug was actually bound to the mitochondria. This binding process could be interfered with by various drugs, including chlorpromazine, reserpine, acetylsalicylate, meprobamate and 1,2,3,4-tetrahydro-9-aminoacridine (THA). The latter drug has been reported by Gershon and Olariu (1960) to be a specific antagonist of the hallucinogenic effects of piperidyl glycollates in man. From this kind of evidence Abood and Biel in 1962 concluded that the action of the piperidyl glycollates was on the mitochondria, probably at the cholinergic receptor sites. Mitochondria have a high phospholipid content and it was suggested that the piperidyl glycollates interacted with the lipid portion of cell membranes. In experiments with frog sartorius muscle Abood and Biel obtained results which led to the conclusion that the drugs affected muscle depolarization by interfering with the movement of ions, notably Ca^{++} and Mg^{++}.

It is possible that all cell membranes, including those of nerve cells, might be affected in a similar manner. There remains the question as to how the effects are initiated. There are at least three possibilities – that the drugs act directly on the membrane or on specific receptors to produce their effects, that they antagonize the effects of naturally occurring neurotransmitter, or that they affect the rate of release or destruction of a naturally occurring neurotransmitter. There seems to be little direct evidence for the first of these possibilities while the second, which seems the most likely, has already been considered above. The third possibility relates to the fact that anticholinergic drugs cause significant decreases in brain content of acetylcholine. This was first discovered for atropine and hyoscine by Giarman and Pepeu (1962). Later the same workers, in 1964, studied four piperidyl glycollates. Two which were hallucinogenic in man caused decreases in brain acetylcholine, while the other two, which were non-hallucinogenic, did not. There is still debate as to the mechanism whereby this decrease is brought about and as to whether it is a primary or a secondary effect. Until this is resolved it is difficult to assess the importance of the effect in the hallucinogenic mode of action of anticholinergic drugs.

CANNABIS

The term cannabis covers a wide variety of products from the Indian hemp *Cannabis sativa.* These products have innumerable names in different parts of the world but basically there are two types of material (Joyce, 1970): the exudate or resin from the flowering tops and leaves, best known as hashish, and the material obtained by chopping the leaves and stalks, best known as marihuana.

The active principle of cannabis was long in doubt but the isolation of Δ^9-tetrahydrocannabinol (XVIII) from marihuana (Mechoulam and Gaoni, 1967), its subsequent synthesis (Petrzilka and Sikemeir, 1967), and the demonstration of its marihuana-like activity in man (Isbell *et al.*, 1967) has led to the belief that this compound, in its *trans* configuration (Δ^9-THC) is responsible, in the main, for hallucinogenic activity. Also active and present in the plant is Δ^8-*trans*-tetrahydrocannabinol (XIX, Δ^8-THC) together with various other, apparently biologically inactive cannabinoids.

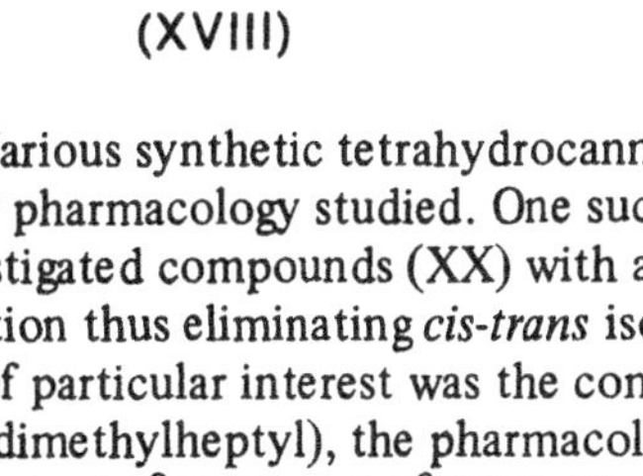

(XVIII)

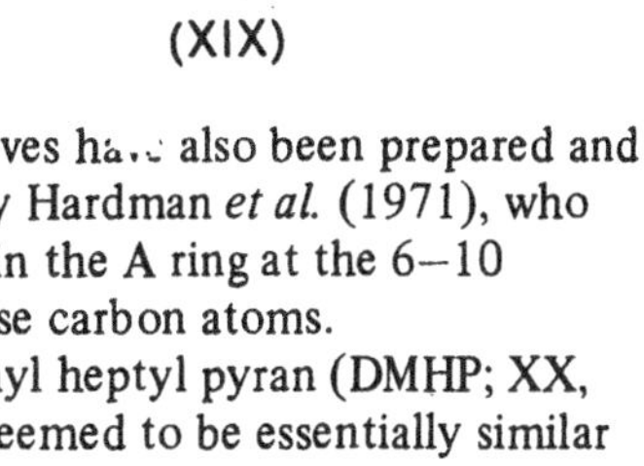

(XIX)

Various synthetic tetrahydrocannabinol derivatives have also been prepared and their pharmacology studied. One such study was by Hardman *et al.* (1971), who investigated compounds (XX) with a double bond in the A ring at the 6–10 position thus eliminating *cis-trans* isomerism at these carbon atoms.

Of particular interest was the compound dimethyl heptyl pyran (DMHP; XX, R = dimethylheptyl), the pharmacology of which seemed to be essentially similar to that of Δ^9 THC and Δ^8 THC. The main general effects noted were central nervous system depression, hypotension, and hypothermia. Although precise

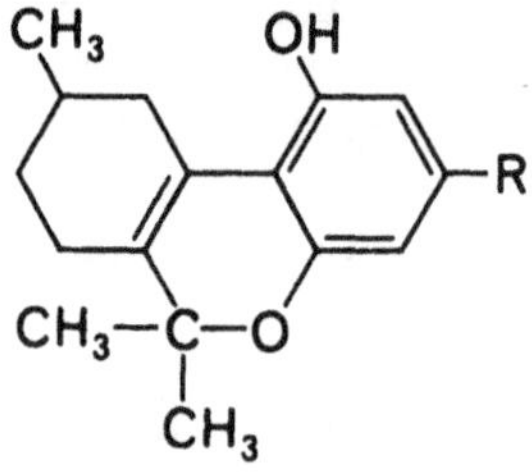

(XX)

quantitative data were not available there was an impression that DMHP was more potent than Δ^9-THC and had a longer duration of action. The hypothermic action of Δ^9-THC had been reported previously by Holtzman *et al.* (1969), who claimed that this action was correlated with elevated brain 5-HT and noradrenaline levels. Elevated levels of 5-HT in the brain after administration of cannabis extract were also reported by Bose *et al.* (1964) but no changes in levels of 5-HT or of catecholamines could be detected by Garattini (1965). This appears to warrant further study.

The central actions of DMHP were reported by Domino *et al.* (1971). The drug had analgesic properties, caused a blockade of conditioned avoidance responses, and produced changes in the electrical activity of the brain which correlated well with gross behavioural effects. Again these effects resembled those reported by others for Δ^9-THC and Δ^8-THC.

Although afferent input appeared to be distorted the blockade of the avoidance response seemed to be due mainly to actions on higher brain centres producing a confusional or depressed state. Neuropharmacological studies suggested that the primary site of action of the drug was in the cerebrum, especially in the secondary association cerebral cortices and related subcortical structures. As with biochemical studies there is obviously the need for more controlled and detailed neuropharmacological and behavioural studies before there can be any clear idea of the mode of action of cannabis.

There have been few controlled human studies with natural preparations of cannabis; in any case difficulties in estimation of the dose and the presence of variable amounts of substances other than THC would make comparative assessment of the results impossible. Even in recent studies with synthetic Δ^9-THC there are difficulties. Hollister (1971) has pointed out that the way in which the material is handled after synthesis may affect the actual dose administered. Since it appears that decarboxylation of the THC acids is necessary before they become biologically active, oral administration of the drug gives variable results since the degree of *in vivo* decarboxylation is variable. Smoking the THC reduces this error since the heat generated decarboxylates most THC acids. However, the amount of material absorbed by smoking is very variable depending on the technique used.

Allowing for these difficulties, the work of Isbell *et al.* (1967) showed that clear effects of Δ^9-THC were obtained with a dose of 120 μg. per kg. by mouth or 50 μg. per kg. by smoking. Very pronounced effects, with perceptual distortions, depersonalization, and visual and auditory hallucinations, resulted from 300–400 μg. per kg. orally or 200–250 μg. per kg. by smoking.

In Hollister's (1971) study the effects of Δ^9-THC and synhexyl (XX, R = nC_6H_{13}) were compared in man when administered orally or by smoking. By mouth synhexyl appeared to have about one-third of the activity of Δ^9-THC whereas by smoking it was less active by a factor of about 3 to 6. Both compounds produced similar effects although those resulting from synhexyl were slower in onset and longer in duration than those from Δ^9-THC.

It was concluded that there were marked objective differences between the effects of Δ^9-THC and of LSD-25. Subjectively, it seemed that Δ^9-THC produced less total impairment of function with more euphoria and dream-like states than LSD-25 at comparable doses and that sedation was commonly seen with Δ^9-THC but not with LSD-25. These conclusions are very similar to those reached by Isbell and Jasinski (1969), who found relatively small differences between the subjective effects of the drugs but whereas LSD-25 increased body temperature and blood pressure and deep tendon reflexes and also dilated pupils, Δ^9-THC had none of these effects. No cross-tolerance could be demonstrated between LSD-25 and Δ^9-THC.

The evidence seems to be very much in favour of different modes of action for LSD-25 and Δ^9-THC, although even less is known concerning the action of the latter than of the former.

METHODS OF EVALUATION OF HALLUCINOGENICS

No attempt will be made here to review the wide variety of methods which have been employed to test for hallucinogenic activity in experimental animals or in man. There are, however, a few general points which are worth making. Many of the effects of these drugs in man are entirely subjective so that considerable reliance has to be placed on the subject himself being able to give accurate descriptions of the effects he experiences. The experimenter working with laboratory animals has to try to detect these tenuous and indefinite effects in animals which may not even be capable of experiencing them. He has, therefore, to resort to indirect or empirical methods.

The indirect approach depends on investigating many facets of the pharmacological activity of individual hallucinogenic drugs, or of related series of drugs, to determine whether any aspect of their pharmacology correlates with, or bears any relationship to, their hallucinogenic activity. This kind of approach, as well as being of potential value in screening, can also give some idea as to the mode of action of the drugs.

In the more empirical approach the procedure is to take a number of hallucinogenic drugs, of different chemical types, and to determine whether they produce any common effect, usually on some aspect of animal behaviour. New drugs affecting the same aspect of behaviour in the same way are then likely to be hallucinogenic in their action also. Though it should not be assumed that common effects necessarily result from common mechanisms of action, nevertheless it may be possible, with further experience, to show that some types of hallucinogens share a final common pathway in their actions.

The aims and objects of workers who are concerned with the evaluation of hallucinogenic drugs in man are somewhat different from those of the laboratory animal experimenter. There will usually be knowledge, or at any rate a suspicion, that the drug has hallucinogenic properties from previous deliberate or accidental human exposures, from the results of animal experiments, or from the fact that chemically closely related structures have this sort of activity. The experimenter will be concerned to categorize, as accurately as possible, the effects of the drug on psychological or psychomotor performance, to determine how closely the effects resemble those seen in the naturally occurring psychoses and to establish whether the drug is likely to be of value in the treatment of any mental condition.

REFERENCES

ABOOD, L. G. (1968), The psychotomimetic glycolate esters. In: *Drugs affecting the Central Nervous System* (ed. BURGER, A.), p. 127. New York: Dekker.

—, and BIEL, J. H. (1962), Anticholinergic psychotomimetic agents, *Int. Rev. Neurobiol.*, **4**, 217–273.

—, OSTFELD, A., and BIEL, J. H. (1958), A new group of psychotomimetic agents, *Proc. Soc. exp. Biol. Med.*, **97**, 483–486.

—, —, — (1959), Structure activity relationships of 3-piperidyl benzilates with psychotogenic properties, *Archs int. Pharmacodyn. Thér.*, **120**, 186–200.

—, and RINALDI, F. (1959), Studies with a tritium labelled psychotomimetic agent, *Psychopharmacologia*, **1**, 117–123.

BALESTRIERI, A. (1957), Cross tolerance between LSD-25 and mescaline. In *Psychototropic Drugs* (ed. GARATTINI, S. and GHETTI, V.), p. 581. New York, Elsevier.

BEBBINGTON, A. and BRIMBLECOMBE, R. W. (1965), Muscarinic receptors in the peripheral and central nervous systems, *Adv. Drug Res.*, **2**, 143–172.

BISHOP, P. O., BURKE, W., DAVIS, R., and HAYHOW, W. R. (1960), Drugs as tools in visual physiology with particular reference to (a) The effects of prolonged disuse and (b) The origin of the electroencephalogram, *Trans. ophthal. Soc. Aust.*, **20**, 50–65.

BOAKES, R. J., BRADLEY, P. B., BRIGGS, I., and DRAY, A. (1970). Antagonism of 5-hydroxytryptamine by LSD-25 in the central nervous system: a possible neuronal basis for the actions of LSD-25, *Br. J. Pharmac. Chemother.*, **40**, 202–218.

BOSE, B. C., SAIFI, A. Q., and BHAGWAT, A. W. (1964), Studies on pharmacological actions of *Cannabis indica* (Linn) Part III, *Archs int. Pharmacodyn. Thér.*, **147**, 291–297.

BOSZORMENYI, Z., DER, P., and NAGY, T. (1959), Observations on the psychotogenic effect of *N,N*-diethyltryptamine: A new tryptamine derivative, *J. ment. Sci.*, **105**, 171–181.

BRADLEY, P. B., and ELKES, J. (1953), The effect of amphetamine and D-lysergic acid diethylamide (LSD-25) on the electrical activity of the brain of the conscious cat, *J. Physiol., Lond.*, **120**, 13P–14P.

—, — (1957), The effect of some drugs on the electrical activity of the brain, *Brain*, **80**, 77–117.

—, and MARLEY, E. (1965), Effect of tryptamine and tryptamine homologues on cerebral electrical activity and behaviour in the cat, *Br. J. Pharmac. Chemother.*, **24**, 659–674.

BRIMBLECOMBE, R. W. (1967), Hyperthermic effects of some tryptamine derivatives in relation to their behavioural activity, *Int. J. Neuropharmac.*, **6**, 423–429.

— (1970), Effects of drugs which interact with central muscarinic receptors. In *Drugs and Cholinergic Mechanisms in the CNS* (ed. HEILBRONN, E., and WINTER, A.), pp. 521–527. Stockholm: Forsvarets Forskningsanstalt.

—, and BUXTON, D. A. (1972). Behavioural actions of anticholinergic drugs. In *Biochemical and Pharmacological Mechanisms Underlying Behaviour* (ed. BRADLEY, P. B., and BRIMBLECOMBE, R. W.), pp. 115–125. Amsterdam: Elsevier.

—, and GREEN, D. M. (1967), Further evidence for cholinergic synapses in the mesodiencephalic activating system, *J. Physiol., Lond.*, **194**, 16P–17P.

—, — (1968), The peripheral and central actions of some anticholinergic substances, *Int. J. Neuropharmac.*, **7**, 15–22.

BROWN, F. C. (1971), *Hallucinogenic Drugs.* Springfield, Ill.: Thomas.
CERLETTI, A., and ROTHLIN, E. (1955), Role of 5-hydroxytryptamine in mental diseases and its antagonism to lysergic acid derivatives, *Nature, Lond.*, **176**, 785–786.
CHOTHIA, C., and PAULING, P. (1969), On the conformations of hallucinogenic molecules and their correlation. *Proc. natn. Acad. Sci. U.S.A.*, **63**, 1063–1070.
COSTA, E., GESSA, G. L., HIRSCH, C., KUNTZMAN, R., and BRODIE, B. B. (1962), On current status of serotonin as a brain neurohormone and in action of antireserpine drugs, *Ann. N.Y. Acad. Sci.*, **96**, 118–130.
CURTIS, D. R., and DAVIS, R. (1962), Pharmacological studies upon neurones of the lateral geniculate nucleus of the cat, *Br. J. Pharmac. Chemother*, **18**, 217–246.
DE JONG, H. H. (1945), *Experimental Catatonia.* Baltimore: Williams and Wilkins.
DOMINO, E. F., HARDMAN, H. F., and SEEVERS, M. H. (1971), Central nervous system action of some tetrahydrocannabinol derivatives, *Pharmac. Rev.*, **23**, 317–336.
DOWNING, D. F. (1962), The chemistry of the psychotomimetic substances, *Q. Rev.*, **16**, 133–162.
EVARTS, E. V. (1957), A review of the neurophysiological effects of lysergic acid diethylamide (LSD) and other psychotomimetic agents, *Ann. N.Y. Acad. Sci.*, **66**, 479–495.
— (1958), Effects of a series of indoles on synaptic transmission in the lateral geniculate nucleus of the cat. In *Progress in Neurobiology III. Psychopharmacology* (ed. PENNES, H. H.) pp. 173–194. New York: Hoeber and Harper.
FABING, H. D., and HAWKINS, J. R. (1956), Intravenous bufotenine injection in the human being, *Science, N.Y.*, **123**, 886–887.
FINKELSTEIN, B. A. (1961), Ditran, a psychotherapeutic advance. A review of one hundred and three cases, *J. Neuropsychiat*, **2**, 144–148.
FREEDMAN, D. X. (1961), Effects of LSD-25 on brain serotonin, *J. Pharmac. exp. Ther.*, **134**, 160–166.
—, and AGHAJANIAN, G. K. (1966), Approaches to the pharmacology of LSD-25, *Lloydia*, **29**, 309–313.
FRIEDHOFF, A. J., and VAN WINKEL, E. (1962), The characteristics of an amine found in urine of schizophrenic patients, *J. nerv. ment. Dis.*, **135**, 550–558.
GADDUM, J. H. (1953), Antagonism between lysergic acid diethylamide and 5-hydroxy-tryptophan, *J. Physiol., Lond.*, **121**, 15P.
GALAMBOS, R. (1960), Studies of the auditory system with implanted electrodes, In *Neural Mechanisms of the Auditory and Vestibular Systems.* (ed. RASMUSSEN, G. L., and WINDLE, W. R.) p. 137. Springfield, Ill.: Thomas.
GARATTINI, S. (1965), Effects of a cannabis extract on gross behaviour. In *Hashish, its Chemistry and Pharmacology* (ed. WOLSTENHOLME, G. E., and KNIGHT, J.) pp. 70–78. London: Churchill.
GERSHON, S., and OLARIU, J. (1960), JB329. A new psychotomimetic, its antagonism by tetrahydroaminoacrin and its comparison with LSD, Mescaline and Sernyl, *J. Neuropsychiat.*, **1**, 283–292.
GESSNER, P. K., GODSE, D. D., DRULL, A. H., and McMULLAN, J. M., (1968), Structure-activity relationships among 5-methoxy-N:N-dimethyltryptamine, 4-hydroxy-N:N-dimethyltryptamine (psilocin) and other substituted tryptamines, *Life Sci.*, 7, 267–277.

GIARMAN, N. J., and PEPEU, G. (1962), Drug-induced changes in brain acetylcholine. *Br. J. Pharmac. Chemother.*, **19**, 226–234.

—, — (1964), The influence of centrally acting cholinolytic drugs on brain acetylcholine levels. *Ibid.*, **23**, 123–130.

GREEN, D. M. (1972), Personal communication.

—, and ALDOUS, F. A. B. (1972), The effect of anticholinergic drugs, chlorpromazine and LSD-25 on evoked potentials, EEG and behaviour. In *Biochemical and Pharmachological Mechanisms Underlying Behaviour*, (ed. BRADLEY, P. B., and BRIMBLECOMBE, R. W.), pp. 143–157. Amsterdam: Elsevier.

HARDMAN, H. F., DOMINO, E. F., and SEEVERS, M. H. (1971), General pharmacological actions of some synthetic tetrahydrocannabinol derivatives, *Pharmac. Rev.*, **23**, 295–315.

HERZ, A. (1963), Excitation and inhibition of cholinoceptive brain structures and its relationship to pharmacological induced behaviour changes, *Int. J. Neuropharmac.*, **2**, 205–216.

HOFMANN, A. (1960), Psychotomimetics: chemical, pharmacological and medical aspects. *Svensk. kem. Tidskr.*, **72**, 723–747.

—, FREY, A. J., OTT, H., PETRIZILKA, T., and TROXLER, F. (1958), Kanstitutionsaufklarung und Sythese von Psilocybin, *Experientia*, **14**, 397–399.

HOLLISTER, L. E. (1961), Clinical, biochemical and psychologic effects of psilocybin, *Archs int. Pharmacodyn., Thér.*, **130**, 42–52.

— (1971), Actions of various marihuana derivatives in man, *Pharmac. Rev.*, **23**, 349–357.

HOLTZMAN, D., LOVEL, R. A., JAFFE, J. J., and FREEDMAN, D. X. (1969), 1-Δ^9-tetrahydro-cannabinol: neurochemical and behavioural effects in the mouse, *Science, N.Y.*, **163**, 1464–1467.

INCH, T. D. (1972), Chemical and stereochemical aspects of behavioural studies. In *Biochemical and Pharmacological Mechanisms Underlying Behaviour* (ed. BRADLEY, P. B., and BRIMBLECOMBE, R. W.), pp. 59–64. Amsterdam: Elsevier.

ISBELL, H. (1967), Discussion on the psychoactive action of various tryptamine derivatives. In *Ethnopharmacologic Search for Psychoactive Drugs* (ed. EFRON, D. H., HOLMSTEDT, B., and KLINE, N. S.) p. 374. Public Health Service Publication No. 1645.

—, and JASINSKI, D. (1969), A comparison of LSD-25 with (–) Δ^9-trans tetrahydrocannabinol (THC) and attempted cross tolerance between LSD and THC, *Psychopharmacologia*, **18**, 108–117.

—, GORODETSKY, C. W., JASINSKI, D., CLAVSSEN, V., VON SPULAK, F., and KORTE, F. (1967), Effects of 1-Δ^9-trans-tetrahydrocannabinol in man, *Ibid.*, **1**, 20–28.

JOYCE, C. R. B. (1970), Cannabis, *Br. J. Hosp. Med.*, **4**, 162–165.

KEY, B. J. (1965a), The effects of drugs on discrimination and sensory generalisation of auditory stimuli in cats, *Psychopharmacologia*, **2**, 352–363.

— (1965b), Effect of lysergic acid diethylamide on potentials evoked in the specific sensory pathway, *Br. med. Bull.*, **21**, 30–35.

LEONARD, B. E., and TONGE, S. R. (1969), The effects of some hallucinogenic drugs upon the metabolism of noradrenaline, *Life Sci.*, **8**, 815–825.

LIPMAN, V. C. (1967), Comparison of anticholinergic potency to psychotomimetic action of glycolate esters, *Proc. Soc. exp. Biol. Med.*, **126**, 172–176.

MARRAZZI, A. S. (1960), Methodological problems in neuropharmacologic research. In *Recent Advances in Biological Research* (ed. WORTIS, J.), pp. 379–401. New York: Grune and Stratton.
—, and HART, E. R. (1953), Comparison of the effect on evoked cortical synaptic response of mescaline, amphetamine and adrenaline. *Electroenceph. clin. Neurophysiol.*, **5**, 317–318.
MECHOULAM, R., and GAONI, Y. (1967), Absolute configuration of Δ^1-tetrahydrocannabinol, the major active constituent of hashish, *Tetrahedron Lett.*, **12**, 1109–1111.
PERETZ, D. I., SMYTHIES, J. R., and GIBSON, W. C. (1955), A new hallucinogen: 3,4,5-trimethoxyphenyl-β-aminopropane, *J. ment. Sci.*, **101**, 317–329.
PERRY, T. L., HANSENS, S., MACDOUGALL, L., and SCHWARZ, C. D. (1966). Urinary amines in chronic schizophrenia. *Nature, Lond.*, **212**, 146–148.
PETRZILKA, T., and SIKEMEIR, C. (1967), Components of hashish II. Synthesis of (–) $\Delta^{6,1}$-3,4-transtetrahydrocannabinol and (±) $\Delta^{6,1}$-3,4-trans-tetrahydrocannabinol, *Helv. chim. Acta*, **50**, 1416–1419.
PURPURA, D. P. (1956), Electrophysiological analysis of psychotogenic drug action, *Archs Neurol. Psychiat.*, **75**, 122–133, 134–143.
RINALDI, F., and HIMWICH, H. E. (1955), Frenquel corrects certain cerebral electrographic charges, *Science, N.Y.*, **122**, 198–199.
ROBINSON, T. (1968). *The Biochemistry of Alkaloids*, p. 77. New York: Verlag.
ROSENBERG, D. E., ISBELL, H., MINER, E. J., and LOGAN, C. R. (1964), The effect of N,N-dimethyltryptamine in human subjects tolerant to lysergic acid diethylamide, *Psychopharmacologia*, **5**, 217–227.
—, WOLBACH, A. B., MINER, E. J., and ISBELL, H. (1963), Observations on direct and cross tolerance with LSD and d-amphetamine in man, *Ibid.*, **5**, 1–15.
SHULGIN, A. T. (1970), Chemistry and structure-activity relationships of the psychotomimetics. In *Psychotomimetic Drugs* (ed. EFRON, D. H.), pp. 21–38. New York: Raven Press.
—, SARGENT, T., and NARANJO, C. (1966), Role of 3,4-dimethoxyphenethyl-amine in schizophrenia, *Nature, Lond.*, **212**, 1606–1607.
—, —, — (1969), Structure-activity relationships of one-ring psychotomimetics, *Ibid.*, **221**, 537–541.
SNYDER, S. H., and RICHELSON, E. (1970), Steric models of drugs predicting psychedelic activity. In *Psychotomimetic Drugs* (ed. EFRON, D. H.), pp. 43–66. New York: Raven Press.
—, WEINGARTNER, H., and FAILLACE, L. A. (1970), DOET (2,5-dimethoxy-4-ethylamphetamine) and DOM(STP) (2,5-dimethoxy-4-methylameptamine) new psychotropic agents: their effects in man. In *Psychotomimetic Drugs* (ed. EFRON, D. H.) pp. 247–264. New York: Raven Press.
SZARA, S. (1956), Dimethyltryptamine: its metabolism in man; the relation of its psychotic effect to the serotonin metabolism, *Experientia*, **12**, 441–442; *Biochem. Pharmac.*, **8**, 324.
—, and HEARST, E. (1962), the 6-hydroxylation of tryptamine derivatives: a way of producing psychoactive metabolites, *Ann. N.Y. Acad. Sci.*, **96**, 134–141.
TONGE, S. R., and LEONARD, B. E. (1969), The effects of some hallucinogenic drugs upon the metabolism of 5-hydroxytryptamine in the brain, *Life Sci.*, **8**, 805–814.

WHITE, R. P., and CARLTON, R. A. (1963), Evidence indicating central atropine-like actions of psychotogenic piperidyl benzilates. *Psychopharmacologia* (*Berl.*), **4**, 459–471.

WOLBACH, A. B., MINER, E. J., and ISBELL, H. (1962), Comparison of psilocin with psilocybin, mescaline and LSD-25. *Ibid.*, **3**, 219–223.

Anticholinesterases: Some Problems in Understanding Their Effects in Whole Animals

J. M. BARNES
Medical Research Council Toxicology Unit, Carshalton

Physiologically and pharmacologically it is difficult to visualize a neater pattern for a mechanism of poisoning than that produced by anticholinesterases. These substances can poison and kill people and animals including insects. There is the enzyme cholinesterase which the biochemist, coming on a corpse days after death, could persuade to show activity. The physiologist, imbued with the overriding importance and activity of acetylcholine in the functioning of the heart, the peripheral and probably the central nervous system, needed the enzyme to ensure the rapid disappearance of acetylcholine after its depolarizing activity had been fulfilled.

Nature and the synthetic chemist have provided some very active inhibitors of cholinesterase and these substances may be rapidly lethal in small doses. Unfortunately, simple pictures have a habit of getting blurred if one examines them closely and the cholinesterase activity-inhibitor relationship in terms of the response of the whole animal is no exception. This brief contribution will try to highlight some of the anomalies – that is, points demanding some intellectual activity – rather than underline and reiterate all the obvious correlations.

Anticholinesterases fall into two general classes; *carbamates* which react with cholinesterase and carbamylate the protein, and *organophosphorus compounds* which phosphorylate the protein. Both chemical reactions can be shown *in vitro* to have the same effect, namely, to prevent the hydrolysis of acetylcholine by the enzyme.

Forensically the carbamates are interesting because the Calabar bean which contains physostigmine – one of the more toxic carbamates – was used as a substitute for a jury in West Africa when judging cases of witchcraft. While Gaddum (1948) stated that suspects were made to eat the beans and 'if they die, as they usually do, they are considered to have been witches', Goodman and Gilman (1955) give more details. The innocent person with nothing to fear ate the beans rapidly and promptly vomited and then recovered. The guilty person partook of the beans slowly and poisoning rather than emesis resulted. These authors also state that guilt was assumed if the person showed the signs of poisoning by physostigmine and the mortality from poisoning among West African witches remains in my mind in some doubt.

This pharmacological anecdote illustrates two points worth discussing in more detail, namely speed of action in relation to the effects of anticholinesterases and the cause and prevention of death. The very rapid onset of vomiting was certainly noted in recent years by colleagues in Zagreb studying candidate carbamate insecticides by experiments on themselves (Vandekar *et al.*, 1971). A further point is that despite the synthesis of many carbamate anticholinesterases, some with acute toxicity greater than organophosphate insecticides that have caused deaths, the wide use of some of them has not led to any fatal cases of poisoning. However, the carbamates can be associated with dramatic poisoning. The chemist who left a bottle of isolan on a shelf at home nearly caused the death of his housekeeper who knocked it off and wiped up the liquid with a cloth. She rapidly collapsed but also rapidly recovered in hospital after atropine (Thölen and Metzeler, 1955). In another report, three cases of swallowing isolan – presumably suicidally – were not fatal (Lutterotti, 1961). When spraymen in Nigeria applied a candidate carbamate insecticide, 2-*iso*-propylphenyl carbamate, inside houses they collapsed within two hours, as did an entomologist who attempted the completion of the spraying of a house. All recovered rapidly (Vandekar, 1965). With the less toxic 3-*iso*-propoxyphenyl carbamate which has been successfully sprayed inside many houses in some malaria eradication programmes where DDT resistant vectors exist, there have been many episodes where spraymen have had to give up, mainly with severe weakness and sweating. However, with a short rest outside they rapidly recover and may return to continue spraying for the rest of the day (Wright *et al.*, 1969). Special studies of some of these spraymen show that they rapidly develop a considerable reduction of their blood cholinesterase levels but do not necessarily show symptoms. If symptoms do appear it is not possible to link them with additional measurable depression of blood cholinesterase. Thus the margin between disabling signs and symptoms is very small in the case of carbamates, suggesting that the balance between active enzyme and level of acetylcholine at the myoneural junction is very delicate.

With the organophosphorus insecticides the picture is somewhat different. With the more toxic ones like parathion, when signs of poisoning appear after occupational exposure they often proceed remorselessly in the absence of further exposure and may be fatal if treatment is not rigorous and prolonged.

In suicide cases, however, where parathion is swallowed, death is often quite rapid and in a series of these cases studied by Pribilla (1955) the average level of blood cholinesterase activity after death was around 40 per cent of normal. Death in organophosphate poisoning following the classic studies of de Candole and others at Porton many years ago (de Candole *et al.*, 1953) appears to be due to failure of the respiratory centre. This implies that it is the cholinesterase levels in the brain stem that are important. In a recent study on mice poisoned with sarin, Bajgar (1971) showed that the signs of poisoning after different doses could best be correlated with changes in levels of cholinesterase activity in pons and medulla rather than those in other parts of the brain. Furthermore, the amount of cholinesterase varies greatly in different parts of the brain and the proportion inhibited by circulating inhibitor will depend on the concentration of enzyme at the various places (Bajgar, 1972).

In producing acute effects by either carbamates or organophosphates it seems clear that speed of inhibition of the enzyme may be just as important as the degree to which inhibition proceeds, reminding one of Paton's rate hypothesis (Paton, 1961). Thus it was early discovered in patients with myasthenia gravis treated with small repeated doses of organophosphorus compounds that the blood enzyme could be reduced to zero activity without the patients developing symptoms. Tissue levels under these circumstances can only be determined in animal experiments, but these show that animals may survive with 10 per cent of normal brain enzyme activity. If the inhibition is produced fairly rapidly over a few days by putting the inhibitor in the diet, severe signs of poisoning may appear within a few days, but despite the continued feeding of the diet and the continued depression of brain cholinesterase the animals gradually improve and soon appear normal and grow well (Barnes and Denz, 1954). Dubois showed that these animals have become more resistant to acetylcholine and carbachol (Broden and Dubois, 1964). However, under other experimental conditions it appears that the tissues become adapted to the effects of higher concentrations of acetylcholine much more rapidly. If an anaesthetized animal is given a lethal dose of an organophosphate such as paraoxon and revived by artificial respiration, normal breathing is resumed and the animal is now resistant to further doses of inhibitor even while measurable levels of acetylcholine accumulate in the blood (Barnes and Duff, 1954) The isolated rat diaphragm quickly begins to function almost normally again after virtually all cholinesterase has been inhibited but passes through a disordered phase while the inhibition proceeds (Barnes and Duff, 1953). Krivoy and Wills (1956) showed that the perfused cervical ganglion quickly became adapted to levels of acetylcholine in the perfusate that initially completely blocked its activity. It is not easy to fit this evidence of rapid adaption to effects of excess of acetylcholine with the severity of the effects of poisoning by some organophosphorus compounds where this proceeds relatively slowly as with parathion in moderate doses, under conditions of occupational exposure.

Speed of inhibition is clearly important in producing symptoms and even death, but the latter appears to be very much less likely if the rate of inhibition is offset by speedier reactivation of the enzyme. The half-life of monomethyl carbamylated cholinesterase is 30 minutes but that of cholinesterase inhibited by paraoxon is 2–3 days. On the other hand the half-life after inhibition by methyl paraoxon is 1½ hours. It is thus interesting to note that while the acute oral toxicity of methyl parathion to rats is not much less than that of parathion, there have been no reports of occupational fatalities from methyl parathion despite its extensive use. Thus, while the simple picture of death or disability in anticholinesterase poisoning being the result of excess of acetylcholine at sensitive sites is undoubtedly generally correct, it is not always easy to explain in these simple terms the differences in the acute or subacute response of animals to different inhibitors of the enzyme. If we are concerned with factors that decide whether exposure will lead to death or disability and the effects of different forms of therapy, it would be a great help if we knew a little more about the ways in which the delicate balance between enzyme activity, and level of acetylcholine determine the local responses at the periphery and in the central nervous system.

A most striking example of the difficulties in simple explanations is presented by the phenomenon first observed by Koster in 1946 (Koster, 1946). He found that if he gave cats a small dose of physostigmine which itself produced mild signs of poisoning, the animals would then withstand several times the LD_{50} of di-*iso*-propylphosphorofluoridate (DFP) given a few minutes later. Not only did the cats not die but they recovered from the effects of DFP much more rapidly than those not pretreated by physostigmine. If he gave the cats a small dose of atropine enabling them to tolerate somewhat larger doses of physostigmine, he could protect them against nearly 50 lethal doses of DFP. On the other hand if he gave the animals a small dose of DFP they remained more sensitive than normal cats to physostigmine for several days. Many years ago while the Unit was still at Porton, I repeated these observations on rats and found that doses as low as 0·01 mg. per kg.

physostigmine would protect them from lethal doses of tetraethyl pyrophosphate or paraoxon, but not of parathion.

For many years now we have been studying the phenomenon of delayed neurotoxicity in hens produced by DFP. This necessitates the injection of a dose of 1–2 mg. per kg. of DFP and even with repeated doses of atropine the hens are severely affected for 24–48 hours and a few may die. If, however, the hens are given atropine and 0·1 mg. per kg. physostigmine 10 minutes before the DFP they will display no toxic signs whatsoever until 10 days later when the ataxia – which we are studying – makes its appearance. I stress the observations on the hens because one appears to have abolished all the acute manifestations of cholinergic poisoning by this procedure and it is now necessary to consider the explanation for the phenomenon of protection put forward by Koster. He suggested that the dose of physostigmine inhibited some of the cholinesterase and that when the DFP was given this part of the cholinesterase was protected and therefore could not react with DFP. Meanwhile the DFP itself rapidly disappeared by hydrolysis, cleavage by other esterases, and binding to other proteins.

The carbamylated esterase with its half-life of 30 minutes then returns to activity which now remains in the absence of any DFP to phosphorylate it. This seems a tidy picture until one tries to visualize the situation soon after the DFP is given. Let us assume that 20 per cent of the cholinesterase is 'protected' from the DFP because it is carbamylated. If it is carbamylated then it is unable to hydrolyse acetylcholine and thus cannot perform its normal function. The rest of the cholinesterase is however exposed to the action of the DFP and become phosphorylated so that the enzyme is inactivated. With 20 per cent carbamylated and 80 per cent phosphorylated, all the enzyme is inactivated and the animal should be dead – or at least ill. In the case of our hens they are not even visibly disturbed.

One explanation suggested is that the partial inhibition of the enzyme by the carbamate leads to some accumulation of acetylcholine which does not disturb the animal because the sensitive sites rapidly adjust to a slight excess of acetylcholine as mentioned above. If this is a valid explanation why does a pretreatment with DFP and presumably a resulting accumulation of acetylcholine make the animal more sensitive rather than less sensitive to physostigmine? The biochemical data indicates that an excess of substrate – acetylcholine – is equally effective in protecting the enzyme from carbamylation or from phosphorylation.

The other possibility is that with the short half-life of the carbamylated cholinesterase, as soon as the merest trace of the enzyme is reactivated so it is immediately protected by acetylcholine; this suggests that the acetylcholine accumulates to some level above the normal virtually non-detectable level. If this is the case why does the animal not display some signs of poisoning even if the effects are not lethal, especially at sites where atropine is not effective? There is no simple explanation of these very reproducible experimental findings, but one is left mystified by the exact situation which determines whether or not there is gross malfunction at a cholinergic synapse or nerve ending. One thing that seems quite certain is that these events reflect a very dynamic situation because the protection by physostigmine is only effective if the phosphorylating agent against which protection is sought disappears quite rapidly from the tissues.

Thus protection against parathion which is relatively persistent cannot be achieved by a régime that protects against the active moiety paraoxon because the latter is continuously released as a result of the metabolism of the parathion.

It is not possible to suggest experimental techniques that will disclose what is happening at the points where acetylcholine is released to depolarize membranes and then removed under conditions which ensure normal function and the slightly different conditions which result in malfunction or even non-function, which if it involves respiration may be fatal.

The effects of anticholinesterases on behaviour also raise questions about the role of acetylcholine. The earliest experiments by Russell and his colleagues (Russell *et al.*, 1961) detected changes in rats chronically exposed to the organophosphorus insecticide demeton only when brain cholinesterase was reduced by 50 per cent or more of normal activity. In acute experiments Glow and Rose (1965) detected effects in rats given almost an LD_{50} of DFP, while Goldberg and Johnson (1964) found behavioural effects in rats given only 1/25th of the LD_{50} of a carbamate.

Men who have had toxic doses of carbamates refer to a striking feeling of weakness and if smaller mammals are similarly affected this factor must be taken into account in any behaviour tests, as, indeed, it was by Glow and Rose. Otherwise it is difficult to believe that as much acetylcholine accumulates in the brains of rats given the smaller doses of carbamates as in those given the organophosphorus compounds.

Claims that men having small quantities of organophosphorus insecticides, insufficient to produce the usual symptoms, would nevertheless show failure in performance were not substantiated by the careful studies of Durham *et al.* (1965). The only likely cause of such things as driving or flying accidents among pesticide applicators appeared to be unilateral miosis with the resulting disturbance of vision.

What seems clear is that determination of the acute mammalian toxicity of compounds by injection may not give a clear picture of the comparative hazards when people are exposed to them under conditions which may lead to different rates of both absorption and inactivation of enzymes, depending in turn on different rates at which tissue concentration of the inhibitor and the substrate are reached at the various sensitive sites.

There is no evidence that the rates of reactivation of a phosphorylated or carbamylated cholinesterase are changed appreciably by acetylcholine concentrations round the enzyme. The factors that must come into play to determine how effective pretreatment with a carbamate will be in protecting an animal against a lethal dose of an organophosphorus compound include the following:

a. The relative affinities of the two inhibitors for the cholinesterase and the relation of these affinities to that of acetylcholine.

b. The speed with which the concentration of the organophosphorate is reduced round cholinesterase at sensitive sites. This depends in turn on (i) its rate of destruction by water, A esterases, oxidative reactions or other means; (ii) its binding to alternative sites; and (iii) whether it is being generated over an appreciable period by metabolism of a precursor.

c. The rates of reactivation of the inhibited cholinesterase.

Because the enzymes of different species behave differently in their reactions with inhibitor and because the metabolism of the inhibitors may also vary, it is quite probable that important species differences in response to protection by carbamates will be observed.

All these factors are amenable to further experimental analysis on the basis of known reactions of cholinesterase with inhibitors which have recently been fully described (Aldridge and Reiner, 1972).

It is perhaps most difficult to try to visualize the speed with which acetylcholine is released and inactivated at a normally functioning synapse and nerve ending and what effects slight variations in such speeds of change may have on function. It is clear that a large part of that cholinesterase normally present is not essential for proper functioning, but it is also obvious that rapid depletions of the enzyme can be disastrous while the changes are taking place. All the evidence is that the margin between death and survival can be very narrow in a rapidly changing situation and it may be extremely hard to predict the effects of slight changes in this dynamic system.

REFERENCES

ALDRIDGE, W. N., and REINER, E. (1972), Enzyme inhibitors as substrates, *Research Monographs, Frontier of Biology*, **26**, Amsterdam: North Holland Publishing Co.

BAJGAR, J. (1971), Influence of tromedoxime and atropine on anticholinesterase activity in some parts of the brain of mice poisoned by isopropylmethyl phosphonofluoridate, *Biochem. Pharmac.*, **20**, 3230–3233.

— (1972), Inhibition of acetyl cholinesterase in different parts of the rat brain by isopropylmethyl-phosphorofluoridate; *in vitro* and *in vivo* experiments, *Ibid.*, **21**, 687–694.

BARNES, J. M., and DENZ, F. A. (1954), The reaction of rats to diets containing octamethyl pyrophosphoramide and *O,O*-diethyl-S-ethylmercaptoethanol thiophosphate, *Br. J. indust. Med.*, **11**, 11–19.

—, and DUFF, J. I. (1953), The role of cholinesterase at the myoneural junction, *Br. J. Pharmac. Chemother.*, **8**, 334–339.

—, — (1954), Acetylcholine production in animals poisoned by diethyl-*p*-nitrophenyl phosphate (Paraoxon), *Ibid.*, **9**, 153–158.

BRODEN, J., and DUBOIS, K. P. (1964), Studies on the mechanism of acquired tolerance by rats to *O,O*-diethyl-S-2-(ethylthio) ethyl phosphorodithioate (Di-syston), *Archs int. Pharmacodyn. Thér.*, **149**, 560–570.

DE CANDOLE, C. A., DOUGLAS, W. N., LOVATT EVANS, C., HOLMES, R., SPENCER, K. E. V., TORRANCE, R. W., and WILSON, K. M. (1953), The failure of respiration in death by anticholinesterase poisoning, *Br. J. Pharmac. Chemother.*, **8**, 466–475.

DURHAM, W. F., WOLFE, H. R., and QUINBY, G. E. (1965), Organophosphorus insecticides and mental alertness, *Archs. envir. Hlth.*, **10**, 55–66.

GADDUM, J. H. (1948). *Pharmacology*, 3rd ed., p. 185 London: Oxford University Press.

GLOW, P. H., and ROSE, S. (1965), Effects of reduced acetylcholinesterase levels on extinction of a conditioned response, *Nature, Lond.*, **206**, 475–477.

GOLDBERG, M. E., and JOHNSON, H. E. (1964), Behavioural effects of a cholinergic stimulant in combination with various psychotherapeutic agents, *J. Pharmac.*, **145**, 367–372.

GOODMAN, L. S., and GILMAN, A. (1955), *The Pharmacological Basis of Therapeutics*, 2nd ed., p. 444. New York: Macmillan.

KOSTER, R. (1946), Synergisms and antagonisms between physostigmine and di-isopropyl fluorophosphate in cats, *J. Pharmac. ext. Ther.*, **88**, 39–46.

KRIVOY, W. A., and WILLS, J. H. (1956), Adaption to constant concentrations of acetylcholine, *J. Pharmac.*, **116**, 220–226.

LUTTEROTTI, A. (1961), Liver damage in poisoning with insecticides, *Medsche. Welt*, **46**, 2430–2433.
PATON, W. D. M. (1961), A theory of drug action based on the rate of drug-receptor combination, *Proc. R. Soc. B*, **154**, 21–69.
PRIBILLA, O. (1955), Poisoning with E605, *Arch. Tox.*, **15**, 210–284.
RUSSELL, R. W., WATSON, R. H. J., and FRANKENHAUSER, M. (1961), Effects of chronic reductions in brain cholinesterase activity on acquisition and extinction of a conditioned avoidance response, *Scand. J. Psychol.*, **2**, 21–29.
THÖLEN, H., and METZELER, E. (1955), Poisoning with insecticides, *Schweiz. med. Wschr.*, **85**, 296–299.
VANDEKAR, M. (1965), Observations on the toxicity of carbaryl, folithion and 3-isopropyl-phenyl-N-methylcarbamate in a village-scale trial in Southern Nigeria, *Bull. Wld Hlth Org.*, **33**, 107–115.
—, PLESTINA, R., and WILHELM, K. (1971), Toxicity of carbamates for mammals, *Ibid.*, **44**, 241–249.
WRIGHT, J. W., FRITZ, R. F., HOCKING, K. S., BABIONE, R., GRATZ, N. G., PAL, R., STILES, A. S., and VANDEKAR, M. (1969), *Ortho*-isopropoxyphenyl methyl carbamate (OMS 33) as a residual spray for the control of anopheline mosquitos, *Ibid.*, **40**, 67–90.

Paraquat Poisoning

K. FLETCHER

Industrial Hygiene Research Group, Imperial Chemical Industries Ltd., Cheshire

Paraquat is a herbicide introduced by Plant Protection Limited for commercial use in this country in 1963; the name strictly refers to the cation. The common paraquat salts are all apparently fully ionized and experiments have shown that the anions, chloride, sulphate, methylsulphate etc., do not affect the toxicity of paraquat. The compound belongs to a group of chemicals, the bipyridyls, and the molecules shown in *Fig.* 1 may be considered typical of the many hundreds that

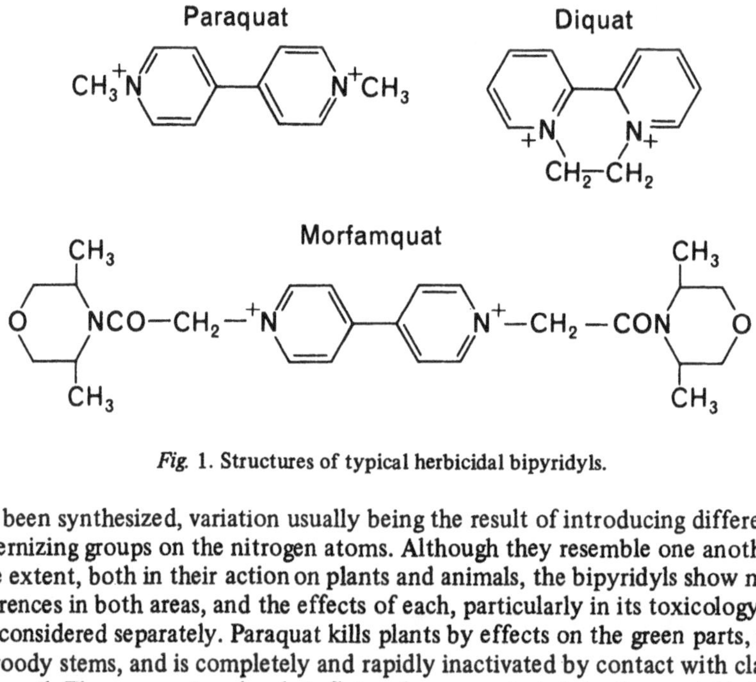

Fig. 1. Structures of typical herbicidal bipyridyls.

have been synthesized, variation usually being the result of introducing different quaternizing groups on the nitrogen atoms. Although they resemble one another to some extent, both in their action on plants and animals, the bipyridyls show major differences in both areas, and the effects of each, particularly in its toxicology, are best considered separately. Paraquat kills plants by effects on the green parts, not on woody stems, and is completely and rapidly inactivated by contact with clay in the soil. The paraquat molecule is flat and can penetrate into the crystal lattice of clay minerals where it is extremely firmly held by physical bonding; in this situation it cannot be attacked by soil organisms which are unable to penetrate the lattice. The only feasible way at present for removing the paraquat is to boil the soil with sulphuric acid and destroy the clay. Paraquat in its bound form is biologically completely inert and has been shown to cause no harm to either plant or animal life. Virtually all soils contain some clay, those that do not being extremely rare, and if paraquat somehow were to be free in the soil, it has been shown that it could be degraded by microorganisms. There is therefore every reason to believe that environmental contamination and a possibly associated toxicological hazard presents no problem with paraquat. These properties enable one to kill weeds on the ground and then plant or seed directly through the killed vegetation and this can, in favourable circumstances, lead to the elimination of ploughing and other traditional cultivation techniques (for a review of the agricultural properties and uses of paraquat see Calderbank (1968)). Because of these properties, paraquat, the best of the bipyridyls, has become widely accepted and is now used in over 130 countries.

Paraquat, for agricultural purposes, is sold primarily as a 20 per cent aqueous solution under the trade name of Gramoxone, although other formulations are in limited use. On the domestic market, paraquat is sold as Weedol, a solid granule, which, until 1971, contained 5 per cent paraquat, but now contains 2·5 per cent paraquat together with 2·5 per cent diquat. During the 10 years of use and in all countries of use, 232 deaths from paraquat poisoning have been reported, about half of these being suicidal. In those cases where we have adequate information all deaths, both suicidal and accidental, have been due to the drinking of concentrated material. (There is an exception to this where a man killed himself by injecting the material (Almog and Tal, 1967).) In the accidental cases swallowing of the material has occurred after it has been put into an unlabelled container in some inappropriate place. Gramoxone has been drunk from a squash bottle in a drinks cupboard, from a beer bottle in a refrigerator, from a whiskey bottle in a larder; children have died after drinking Gramoxone from cordial bottles found in a field or in a farm outhouse or from measuring vessels left unattended. These cases are not exceptional but typical.

Table 1. Paraquat poisoning deaths 1964–1973 (All countries)

	Accident	*Suicide*	*Total**
England and Wales	15	26	49
Scotland	7	6	15
Ireland	22	15	42
W. Germany	9	19	29
Malaysia	8	15	24
Japan	2	10	12
U.S.A.	3	0	3
Other countries (24)	30	18	58
Totals	96	109	232

*The total includes those in which the circumstances of death are unknown.

Table 1 shows the distribution of notified fatal poisoning cases by country, only those countries where several cases have occurred being included. It can be seen that the cases occur predominantly in Western Europe – Ireland, England, and Germany having the most. In the U.S.A., a major user, few cases have occurred. Of the developing territories only Malaysia has a significant number and these are predominantly suicides. There is some tendency for the incidence to reflect total usage, but this is not invariable, and it is noticeable that where one might expect unskilled handling, such as Africa or India, the incidence of poisoning is nil or low. It is apparent that the application of paraquat is not accompanied by any serious risk of poisoning.

The effects of paraquat poisoning were first studied in rats (Clark *et al.*, 1966); changes were seen in these animals which subsequently proved typical of those in other animals and man. The most striking effect is in the lung, the compound initially causing oedema and haemorrhage. If the animal survives this initial phase a fulminating fibrotic process develops and within some 7 to 14 days the lung is a mass of fibrous tissue. Death ensues from anoxia due to a gross impairment of gaseous exchange processes. A detailed description of these changes has now been published elsewhere (Kimbrough and Gaines, 1970). These changes occur whether paraquat is given orally or parenterally, but not when given by inhalation. These dramatic effects in the lung have tended to overshadow the effects of paraquat in other organs, but damage due to paraquat can be demonstrated in the kidneys, liver, and heart. The extent of this damage varies with different species: in the rat, for instance, there is virtually no liver damage and the kidneys are only slightly affected, whereas in the dog all the above organs may be involved. The rabbit appears to be anomalous in that the typical lung changes are not seen in this species (Butler and Kleinerman, 1971).

In man there are now several well investigated reports of the effects of paraquat. The first reaction consequent on the ingestion of Gramoxone is due to its irritancy and usually appears as burning and ulceration of the mouth, oesophagus, and gastrointestinal tract (McDonagh and Martin, 1970; Malone *et al.*, 1971). Diarrhoea is common, sometimes accompanied by blood; curiously vomiting is by no means invariable. The first signs of systemic poisoning are associated with renal damage, usually starting 1–3 days after poisoning, producing an elevated blood urea, reduced creatine clearance, and a diminished urine flow (Oreopoulos, *et al.*, 1968; Gardiner, 1972). The lesion in man is a tubular necrosis similar to that seen in animals. Such effects occur in most cases of poisoning and can be severe, but kidney failure has not been reported as a primary cause of death.

Jaundice as a consequence of damage to the liver is also of common occurrence in man (Fennelly *et al.*, 1971; Grabensee *et al.*, 1971). Post-mortem examination shows a centrilobular necrosis of the liver cells (Bullivant, 1966). The effects on the heart are more varied. Death from heart or circulatory failure has been reported in some instances (Lanzinger *et al.*, 1969; Iff *et al.*, 1971), whereas in many others no apparent defect exists. Post-mortem examination usually does not show any gross lesions, although a patchy degeneration or necrosis of some cardiac muscle fibres may be apparent (Masterson and Roche, 1970). It is possible that the failure of the heart is not entirely due to the direct effect of paraquat on this organ, but is a reflection of the total body damage.

In the majority of cases of poisoning, the above effects, although seriously complicating therapy, seem to be reversible and relatively normal function appears after a few days. The most serious threat to life and the cause of death in most instances is the damage to the lung. In the past, attention has been concentrated on the fibrosis developing after a long delay, rapidly leading to respiratory insufficiency. It is now apparent, however, that damage to the lung occurs early in paraquat poisoning, although this may not be clinically apparent. Yoneyama *et al.* (1969) have described a case of death in one day after a large dose of Gramoxone where lung haemorrhage was present, and von der Hardt and Cardesa (1971) found lung haemorrhage and almost complete loss of the alveolar and bronchiolar epithelium in a woman dying two days after swallowing Gramoxone. Similar findings have also been reported by others (Hargreave *et al.*, 1969; Nagi, 1970).

The more usual case of a delay before lung involvement is clinically apparent, is typified by the reports of Bronkhorst *et al.* (1968), Fennelly *et al.* (1968), McDonagh and Martin (1970), Bony *et al.* (1971), and Grabensee *et al.* (1971), where death was delayed for up to 26 days. In an unreported case death from pulmonary fibrosis occurred 35 days after deliberate ingestion of Gramoxone. Two other cases are of interest in this respect. In the one reported by Matthew *et al.* (1968) at post-mortem fibrosis was seen not only in the patient's own lung, but also in a lung transplanted six days after ingestion. It is, however, possible that the fibrosis was part of a rejection reaction. These authors also stated that although three days prior to the transplant the patient was clinically and radiologically well, tests showed a pattern of deteriorating lung function; this observation has been confirmed (Matthew, 1971). In the case of Almog and Tal (1967), a patient who injected himself with Gramoxone developed signs of paraquat poisoning typical of those after ingestion and died in severe respiratory distress 18 days after injection. The proliferation of the terminal bronchiolar epithelium seen in animals (Clark *et al.*, 1966) was also noted in this case (Herczeg and Reif, 1968).

Unusual pathological findings at post-mortem include adrenal cortical necrosis (Yoneyama *et al.*, 1969; Nagi, 1970), and oedema and haemorrhage of the brain (Lanzinger *et al.*, 1969; Matthew, 1971; Nienhaus and Ehrenfeld, 1971).

The overall results, therefore, in paraquat poisoning by ingestion or injection are those of a compound causing fairly widespread damage, but having its most severe effect and lethal action on the lung. Animals poisoned by inhalation show a different clinical course (Gage, 1968a). In the form of a respirable aerosol★ (mean particle diameter about 5 μm.) paraquat acts similarly to a powerful irritant such as phosgene and the changes in the lung are typical of such effects. Death, at sufficiently high doses, occurs within a short period and animals not dying within this time recover completely; a delayed fibrosis does not occur. It must be emphasized that reported cases of death from paraquat poisoning have been due to swallowing one or other forms of the concentrate. Symptoms following spraying with paraquat have been noted (Guardascione and di Bosco, 1969; Malone *et al.*, 1971), but it should be remembered that paraquat has been used by millions of people, and coincident illness may be expected. The small number of the incidents and their diverse nature lends support to the probability that illness is coincidental with and not caused by paraquat. In a study of Malayan sprayers (Swan, 1969) excretion of very small quantities of paraquat was frequently seen, but over a period of six weeks adverse reactions were limited to minor effects on the skin. Hearn and Keir (1971), investigating 296 sprayers in Trinidad, stated that despite gross exposure of these men no systemic effects were apparent; effects on the finger-nails were, however, reported.

The chemical diagnosis of paraquat poisoning is achieved by analysis of the urine or tissue for paraquat, since paraquat is not metabolized systemically and is excreted unchanged in the urine (Daniel and Gage, 1966). For analysis it can be reduced by dithionite to an intensely coloured free radical which may be estimated colorimetrically by measuring its absorption at 600 nm.

Tompsett and Brown (Matthew *et al.*, 1968) introduced a quick test for paraquat suitable for immediate clinical use. In doubtful cases of poisoning such a test is essential in deciding whether to start intensive therapy since the more accurate laboratory methods are too time-consuming. In this method sodium dithionite and sodium hydroxide are added to urine which is observed for the development of a

★Such aerosols are not produced by agricultural equipment, where the particle size is mostly in excess of 50 μm.

blue colouration; sensitivity is around 1 μg. per ml. A slightly more complicated, but still fast, method has been given by Sharp *et al.* (1972) with detection limits of 0·2 μg. per ml. For small quantities of paraquat, use can be made of ion-exchange resins to concentrate the cation when the sensitivity can be as high as 5 μg. per 100 ml. (Beyer, 1970; Tompsett, 1970). This method is time-consuming, but is quantitative and can detect either those cases where small amounts have been ingested or where analysis is done several days after poisoning.

The excretion of most of the paraquat absorbed systemically is rapid. Daniel and Gage (1966) using ^{14}C-labelled paraquat in rats showed that after subcutaneous injection 90–100 per cent of the dose was recovered in urine within two days. On the basis of this and similar results it was assumed that toxicologically significant amounts of paraquat were not retained and caused paraquat to be called a 'hit and run compound' (Barnes, 1968). Experience of poisoning in man, however, shows that the situation is more complex.

There is very little knowledge of paraquat excretion in human cases in the very early period after paraquat ingestion. In animals Daniel and Gage (1966) showed that about 75 per cent of the compound is not absorbed after oral administration and is excreted in the faeces, and also that 90 per cent of what is absorbed is excreted in the urine within two days. In man, however, it has now been shown that the excretion of paraquat continues for many days. In the first day of analysis the amount of paraquat is comparatively large, and rapidly declines on subsequent days to a lower level, but the 'tail' of excretion is prolonged. The amounts present in this tail are small and represent only a few percent of the total urinary excretion. In the case of Hensel and Durr (1971), of approximately 400 mg. excreted in total, 350 were present in the urine of the first day. The prolonged excretion has now been reported in several cases (Tompsett, 1970; Beebeejaun *et al.*, 1971; Fisher *et al.*, 1971; Grabensee *et al.*, 1971), and must be presumed to be typical. It is of interest that in most cases where the excretion has been followed, a small peak in the amount of paraquat occurs around the ninth day after poisoning. The significance of this is not clear; it may represent the effect of a recovery of kidney function or possibly a release of retained paraquat by the tissues.

The analysis of blood is of little value since paraquat can seldom be detected after about 24 hours, but paraquat may be found in a variety of tissues after death. Sharp *et al.* (1972) have made a detailed study in the rat and found, after an initial period of four hours, that the highest concentration of paraquat was in the lung, with the kidney and liver containing rather less; the half-life in these tissues was about 56 hours and about 50 hours in the lung. Muscle contained low concentrations of paraquat with a half-life of 4–5 days and could therefore, at a late stage, constitute a major pool of paraquat. In man no obvious accumulation of paraquat in the lung has been shown. At day 4 Hall and Carson (1970) reported kidney to contain 5·8 μg. per g. with 1·6, 1·4, and 0·6 in lung, spleen, and liver respectively; at 8 days Lanzinger *et al.* (1969) found kidney and muscle to contain the greatest concentration (1·76 and 1·52 μg. per g.), whilst liver, lung, and spleen were less (0·9–1·0 μg. per g.). Ten days after ingestion Tompsett (1970) could not detect paraquat in lung tissue whilst finding 0·2–0·9 μg per g. in liver, kidney, and muscle, When death occurred 26 days after poisoning Grabensee *et al.* (1971) found 0·19 and 0·25 μg. per g. in the heart and liver and 0·14 μg. per g. in the lung. Results of analyses in this laboratory in several unreported cases also give similar figures. It is therefore apparent that paraquat can be detected in tissues for a long period after poisoning, and that the distribution is fairly general, with no greater concentrations in the most severely affected tissues.

The lethal dose of paraquat in man has been the subject of much speculation. Lanzinger *et al.* (1969) quote an 'LD_{50}' of 4 mg. per kg. and speculate that it may be even less; this has been quoted by others as the oral LD_{50} (Hargreave *et al.*, 1969). This figure is, however, based on a single case of poisoning by the injection of 1 ml. of Gramoxone (Herczeg and Reif, 1968). Paraquat is known to be relatively poorly absorbed in rats (Daniel and Gage, 1966) and in our own experiments the disparity between the oral and intraperitoneal LD_{50}'s in other species would tend to show that this is a general phenomenon. In man Grabensee *et al.* (1971) found a high excretion in the faeces, and figures for urinary excretion are far lower than the estimates of the dose taken, so that it is reasonable to suppose that in man also, only a fraction of a swallowed dose is absorbed systemically; our original guess of about 5 per cent (Conning *et al.*, 1969) may still be correct.

The use of animal data to predict a lethal dose for man is not particularly helpful. *Table* 2 shows that the oral LD_{50} in a variety of species is very variable. Some slight correlation with body weight can be seen and this might suggest an LD_{50} for man of around 50 mg. per kg. There are, however, obvious anomalies, perhaps the most striking being the difference in LD_{50} between the rabbit and the hare.

Table 2. Oral LD_{50} of paraquat in various animals

Species	*Body weight (g.)*	*LD_{50} (mg. per kg.)*
Mouse	30	104 (90–120)
Rat	175	130 (110–160)
Guinea pig	400	30 (22–41)
Rabbit	2,500	126 (69–183)
Cat	2,500	35 (27–46)
Hare	3,000	35
Monkey	5,500	75
Dog	12,000	25–50
Sheep	25,000	65
Cow	150,000	35–60

In cases of human poisoning it is seldom that the dose is known with even approximate accuracy, such phrases as 'a mouthful' or 'a sip' being used. The situation is further complicated by the patient spitting out or vomiting some of the material. There are, however, a few cases where a good estimate of dose has been obtained. In the case of Fisher *et al.* (1971) 10 ml. Chevron Dual (equivalent to Gramoxone) was swallowed and the patient recovered, despite the absence of treatment for some six days; similarly Iff *et al.* (1971) reported recovery in a 16-year-old boy after 10–15 ml. of 30 per cent paraquat solution. Two remarkable cases are those of Grundies *et al.* (1971) where the dose was 50 ml., with vomiting, but recovery ensued with treatment, and Malone *et al.* (1971) where a 35-year-old man survived 4 oz. (110 ml.).

Against these cases may be set those where death ensued: 30 ml., vomited (Hensel and Durr, 1971), 20 ml. (Matthew, 1971), 10 ml. (Nienhaus and Ehrenfeld, 1971), a teaspoon (?5–10 ml) (Fennelly *et al.*, 1968; Masterson and Roche, 1970).

Cases of poisoning by Weedol have also been reported. In a 32-year-old man 45 g. (equivalent to 2·5 g. paraquat) was survived (Kerr *et al.*, 1968) as was 10 g. (0·5 g. paraquat) in a 2-year-old child (McDonagh and Martin, 1970). Lloyd (1969) reports survival in three children eating 60 g. between them. Death occurred after

160 g. (8 g. paraquat) (Hall and Carson, 1970). We have also been told of a 23-year-old girl dying, after prolonged illness, after taking 20 g. (1 g. paraquat).

If 10 ml. of Gramoxone is taken to be the probable lethal dose this would contain 2 g. of paraquat and in a 60-kg. man would give a lethal amount as just over 30 mg. per kg. paraquat. The total evidence therefore would suggest that the LD_{50} to man of paraquat is about 30 mg. per kg.

The implication, from a history of taking a mouthful and spitting it out, that the lethal dose of Gramoxone is considerably less than indicated above, is difficult to substantiate. Patients giving this account have both died (Bullivant, 1966; Oreopoulos *et al.*, 1968; Heyndrickx *et al.*, 1969; Lanzinger *et al.*, 1969; Tompsett, 1970) and recovered (McKean, 1968; Mracek and Krch, 1969; Grabensee *et al.*, 1971; Malone *et al.*, 1971). It is extremely difficult to avoid swallowing at least some of a liquid which has been taken into the mouth in the mistaken belief that it is innocuous and it is not unreasonable to suppose that in this circumstance 10 ml. can be swallowed; where available, the urinary excretion figures suggest this to be so.

The treatment of paraquat poisoning is at present directed toward the elimination of the material from the body. It has been shown (Clark, 1971) that the mineral adsorbents, Bentonite and Fullers Earth, can remove paraquat very efficiently from the stomach, but this usefulness is confined to the first hour after ingestion. After absorption, treatment is designed to help elimination. Ferguson (1971) has shown that paraquat is freely filtered by the renal glomeruli, but is reabsorbed to some extent in the proximal tubule. Forced diuresis appears to be the treatment of choice, heroic quantities of fluid, up to 30 litres per day being used with success (Grundies *et al.*, 1971). Although these latter authors show that paraquat is freely dialysable, experience with haemodialysis has been disappointing. After 24 hours paraquat is present in blood usually at concentrations undetectable chemically (Sharp *et al.*, 1972) and dialysis will remove little if any. The fact that in these circumstances very appreciable quantities are removed by the kidneys probably reflects the vastly greater rate of blood-flow through these organs.

Immunosuppressive agents and cytotoxic drugs have been used for treatment, but their effectiveness is questionable (Fennelly *et al.*, 1971; Malone *et al.*, 1971). Certainly no consistent response seems to be obtained with their use. Oxygen is quite definitely contraindicated (Matthew, 1971; Nienhaus and Ehrenfeld, 1971; Fisher *et al.*, 1972).

There is at present no substance known to have an antidotal effect in paraquat poisoning. In this laboratory we have examined many compounds for this property, usually on the basis of some hypothesis about the mechanism of toxic action (*Table* 3); without exception these compounds have shown no indication of the required effect. Despite the lack of a specific antidote, an attribute which paraquat shares with the great majority of chemicals in daily use, it is clear that paraquat ingestion is by no means inevitably fatal, even after the appearance of clinical evidence of lung damage. Of the 97 cases recorded in the literature, 29 are of recovery, and in the records kept in this laboratory there are a further 63. (In many of these unreported cases the dose was trivial and would not be expected to lead to symptoms, but on the criteria given above, about half might be classed as serious poisoning.) Recovery seems to be substantially complete, although in one or two cases some residual lung impairment has been reported (Malone *et al.*, 1971; Mracek and Krch, 1969). With a recognition of the problem and the evolution of forms of treatment, the rate of survival would now seem to be higher.

Table 3. Effect of various compounds used as possible antidotes to paraquat poisoning. Groups of 5–10 rats were given a lethal amount of paraquat usually as a single oral dose, but in some instances by incorporation in the diet. The 'antidote' was given by injection. The effectiveness of the antidote was assessed by comparing the group given the antidote with a similar group given paraquat only.

	Compound	*Effect*
Free radical scavengers	2-mercaptoethylamine hydrochloride	Increased mortality
	2-aminoethylisothiouronium bromide	Increased mortality
	Dimethylsulphoxide	Increased mortality
	Cysteamine	No effect
	γ-tocopherol	Some protective action when given before paraquat, none after
Anti-inflammatory	Cortisone	No effect
	Prednisolone	Slight delay in death
	Butazolidine	Slight delay in death
	Chlorpromazine	No effect
Immunosuppressive drugs	Azathiaprine	No effect
	Busulphan	No effect
	Chlorambucil	No effect
Complexing agents	Sodium tetraphenyl borate	Increased mortality
	Sodium amsonate	No effect
Miscellaneous	Trasylol	No effect
	Promethazine hydrochloride	No effect
	Indomethacin	No effect
	Aspirin	No effect
	Calcium EDTA	No effect
	Riboflavin	No effect
	Phenazine	Increased mortality
	100 per cent O_2	Increased mortality
	10 per cent O_2	No effect
	Galactose	No effect
	Theophylline	Increased mortality
	Salbutamol	Increased mortality
	Dibenyline	Increased mortality
	Duramorph	Increased mortality

The biochemical process by which paraquat produces its toxic effects is unknown; possibly the reduction of paraquat to a free radical is involved. Michaelis and Hill (1933) showed many years ago that powerful reducing agents produced a stable free radical and under the name of methyl viologen, paraquat has been used as a redox indicator. The scheme of reactions of *Fig.* 2 can be shown to occur in biological systems. In plants the reduction of paraquat to the radical ion is brought about by photosystem 1, followed by a spontaneous reaction with oxygen to give the O_2^- radical ion and regenerated paraquat. The O_2^- then reacts either spontaneously or enzymatically to give oxygen and hydrogen peroxide, which latter is considered to be the immediate toxic agent in plants (Calderbank, 1968; Dodge, 1971). Similar reactions can occur in animals. Gage (1968b) has shown that flavo-enzymes from rat liver will reduce paraquat to the radical and the subsequent reactions outlined above may be expected to follow. The redox potential of the reduction of paraquat to paraquat radical is –446 mV. and in the isolated enzyme system the amount of radical produced is small. Experiments using pulse radiolysis

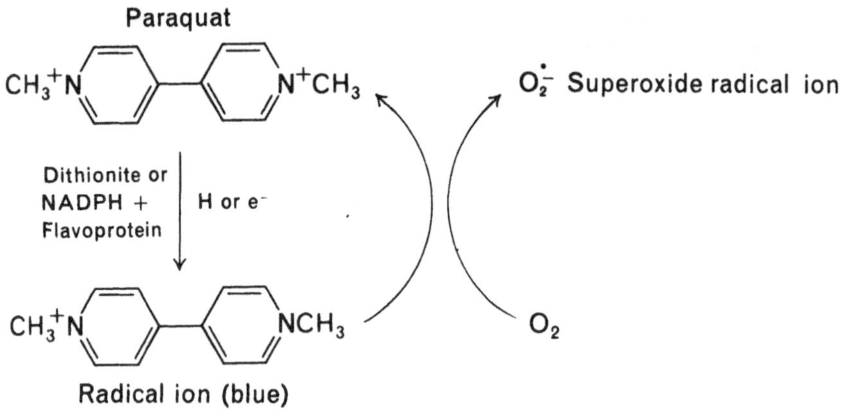

Fig. 2. Reduction and reoxidation of paraquat.

(Farrington, 1971) have shown that the reaction between paraquat radical and O_2 is extremely fast (rate constant in free solution $6{\cdot}5 \times 10^8$ litres per mole sec.) so that the life-time of paraquat radical is very short – of the order of one microsecond with a correspondingly limited diffusion range. The O_2^- radical ion is a normal product of biological processes and the enzyme superoxide dismutase specifically catalyses its rapid removal (McCord and Fridovich, 1969). It would appear then that if these radicals are involved in paraquat toxicity they act at very low concentrations close to the site of production, and the hypothesis that it is paraquat itself that is the direct toxic species must still be tenable. From the prolonged urinary excretion in man and the occurrence of tissue residues many days after ingestion, it must be inferred that tissue binding occurs but the significance of this is not known; it may be a non-specific binding to acidic polymers.

The presence of small quantities of bound paraquat may be relevant to the development of fibrotic reactions in the lung. The case of Matthew *et al.* (1968) would tend to support this view and Styles and Conning (1969) have shown not only that the fibroblast, in contrast to the alveolar macrophage, is relatively resistant to paraquat, but is stimulated into division in the presence of low concentrations. Against this, we have shown (unpublished observations) that small quantities of paraquat producing measurable tissue concentrations can be fed to animals for prolonged periods with no adverse effect, and other organs accumulating as high or higher concentrations than the lung show no fibrosis. In view of the massive damage to the lung known to occur soon after ingestion the fibrosis may well be the normal formation of scar tissue after injury.

Manktelow (1967) introduced the idea that paraquat interfered specifically with the formation of pulmonary surfactant and this was taken up by others (Fisher and Clements, 1969; Robertson *et al.*, 1971). Fletcher and Wyatt (1970) disputed these results on the basis of lipid analysis in rat lungs and later (Fletcher and Wyatt, 1972) found no difference in the dipalmitoyl lecithin content of the lung of paraquat-poisoned mice and controls.

Electron microscopic studies of the effects of paraquat have been made both in animals and man. Vijeyaratnam and Corrin (1971) considered that in rats the major effects of paraquat were produced on the alveolar epithelial tissue, the endothelium being relatively little affected. These effects were produced early after an intraperitoneal injection of paraquat, marked changes occurring within 24 hours leading to complete loss of epithelium after three days. Similar findings were seen by Wasan and McElligott (1972). In the lungs of mice, Fowler and Brooks (1971). found early endothelial cell swelling and damage to alveolar epithelial type A cells, although the type B cells were relatively unaffected, reminiscent of the earlier work reported in rats by Kimbrough and Gaines (1970). Modee *et al.* (1972) showed early capillary engorgement and interstitial oedema followed in 24 hours by mitochondrial degeneration and cytoplasmic vacuolization in various cell types with desquamation of necrotic alveolar epithelial cells at 48 hours. Essentially similar processes were seen in man (Toner *et al.*, 1970) and these authors point out the similarity of the changes to those seen in oxygen poisoning. Fowler and Brooks (1971) studied changes in the proximal convoluted tubules of mice given paraquat and found an increase in the amount of smooth endoplasmic reticulum and the presence of lipid-containing cytosomes. None of these studies has shown paraquat to attack unequivocally a specific cell or cellular constituent, although it would seem that epithelial cells, particuarly in the lung, are preferentially damaged. It is not known whether these cells contain higher concentrations of paraquat than others, nor whether their proximity to the high oxygen tensions of the alveoli is significant.

The circumstances surrounding paraquat poisoning are in some respects peculiar. Although there are many agricultural chemicals of greater intrinsic toxicity, the relatively high oral toxicity of paraquat has led to accidental fatal poisoning, because in virtually all cases concentrated solutions have been drunk from apparently innocuous bottles. In most countries of use, solutions of paraquat are recognized as poisons by the authorities and are labelled as such. Nevertheless, perhaps because of the general usefulness and properties of the material, persons requiring small quantities pour it into unlabelled bottles and it is thereafter that accidents occur. Whilst in comparison with other forms of accidental poisonings those from paraquat are relatively few in number, they should be wholly preventable. Suitable labelling and formulation can help towards this, but only by the elimination of the few cases of irresponsible handling will these unnecessary tragedies cease.

REFERENCES

ALMOG, C., and TAL. E. (1967), Death from paraquat after subcutaneous injection, *Br. med. J.*, **3**, 721.

BARNES, J. M. (1968), Poisons that hit and run, *New Scient.*, **38**, 619–620.

BEEBEEJAUN, A. R., BEEVERS, G., and ROGERS, W. N. (1971), Paraquat poisoning – prolonged excretion, *Clin. Tox.*, **4**, 397–408.

BEYER, R. H. (1970), Analytical determination and toxicity of paraquat (Gramoxone), *Dt. Apothztg.*, **110**, 633–635.

BONY, D., FAVAREL-GARRIGUES, J. C., CLEDES, J., CAMBEILH, J., and CASTAING, R. (1971), Paraquat poisoning, *Eur. J. Tox.*, **4**, 406.

BRONKHORST, F. B., VAN DAAL, J. M., and TAN, H. D. (1968), Fatal outcome of a case of paraquat (Gramoxone) poisoning, *Ned. Tijdschr. Geneesk.*, **112**, 310–313.

BULLIVANT, C. M. (1966), Accidental poisoning by paraquat: report of two cases in man, *Br. med. J.*, **1**, 1272–1273.

BUTLER, C., and KLEINERMAN, J. (1971), Paraquat in the rabbit, *Br. J. ind. Med.*, **28**, 67–71.

CALDERBANK, A. (1968), The bipyridilium herbicides, *Adv. Pest Control*, **8**, 127–235.

CLARK, D. G. (1971), Inhibition of the absorption of paraquat from the gastrointestinal tract by adsorbents, *Br. J. ind. Med.*, **28**, 186–188.

—, McELLIGOTT, T. F., and WESTON HURST, E. (1966), The toxicity of paraquat, *Ibid.*, **23**, 126–132.

CONNING, D. M., FLETCHER, K., and SWAN, A. A. B. (1969), Paraquat and related bipyridyls, *Br. med. Bull.*, **25**, 245–249.

DANIEL, J. W., and GAGE, J. C. (1966), Absorption and excretion of diquat and paraquat in rats, *Br. J. ind. Med.*, **23**, 133–136.

DODGE, A. D. (1971), The mode of action of the bipyridylium herbicides, paraquat and diquat, *Endeavour*, **30**, 130–135.

FARRINGTON, J. A. (1971), In *Proceedings 1st European Biophysics Congress*, (ed. by BRODS, E., LOCKER, A., and SPRINGER-DEDERER, H.) pp. 511–515. Vienna: Weiner Medizinischen Akademie.

FENNELLY, J. J., FITZGERALD, M. X., and FITZGERALD, O. (1971), Recovery from severe paraquat poisoning following forced diuresis and immunosuppressive therapy, *J. Irish. med. Ass.*, **64**, 69–71.

—, GALLAGHER, J. T., and CARROLL, R. J. (1968), Paraquat poisoning in a pregnant woman, *Br. med. J.*, **3**, 722–723.

FERGUSON, D. M. (1971), Renal handling of paraquat, *Br. J. Pharmac. Chemother.*, **42**, 636P.

FISHER, A. B., FRANK, R., and FISHER, H. K. (1972), In *Environmental Factors in Respiratory Disease* (ed. LEE, D. H. K.), pp. 99–102. London and New York: Academic Press.

FISHER, H. K., and CLEMENTS, J. A. (1969), Effects of the herbicide paraquat on mechanical properties of rat lungs, *Fedn Proc. Fedn Am. Socs. exp. Biol.*, **28**, 526.

—, HUMPHRIES, M., and BAILS, R. (1971), Recovery from renal and pulmonary damage, *Ann. intern. Med.*, **75**, 731–736.

FLETCHER, K., and WYATT, I. (1970), The composition of lung lipids after poisoning with paraquat, *Br. J. exp. Path.*, **51**, 604–610.

—, — (1972), The action of paraquat on the incorporation of palmitic acid into dipalmitoyl lecithin in mouse lungs, *Ibid.*, **53**, 225–230.

FOWLER, B. A., and BROOKS, R. E. (1971), Effects of the herbicide paraquat on the ultrastructure of mouse kidney, *Am. J. Path.*, **63**, 505–512.

GAGE, J. C. (1968a), Toxicity of paraquat and diquat aerosols generated by a size-selective cyclone: effect of particle size distribution, *Br. J. ind. Med.*, **95**, 304–314.

— (1968b), The action of paraquat and diquat on the respiration of liver cell fractions, *Biochem. J.*, **109**, 757–761.

GARDINER, A. J. S. (1972), Pulmonary oedema in paraquat poisoning, *Thorax*, **27**, 132–136.

GRABENSEE, B., VELTMANN, G., MURTZ, R., and BORCHARD, F. (1971), Paraquat poisoning, *D. med. Wschr.*, **96**, 498–506.

GRUNDIES, H., KOLMAR, D., and BENNHOLD, I. (1971), Paraquat poisoning, *Ibid.*, **96**, 588–589.

GUARDASCIONE, J., and DI BOSCO, M. M. (1969), Toxicity of the dipyridyl herbicides paraquat to workers, *Folia med., Napoli*, **52**, 728–738.

HALL, R. A., and CARSON, E. D. (1970), Fatal paraquat poisoning, *Bull. int. Ass. Forensic Tox.*, **7**, 5.

HARGREAVE, T. B., GRESHAM, G. A., and KARAYANNOPOULOS, S. (1969), Paraquat poisoning, *Postgrad. med. J.*, **45**, 633–635.

HEARN, C. E. D., and KEIR, W. (1971), Nail damage in spray operators exposed to paraquat, *Br. J. ind. Med.*, **28**, 399–403.

HERCZEG, E., and REIF, A. (1968), Changes in the lung in fatal cases of paraquat poisoning, *Zentbl. allg. Path. path. Anat.*, **111**, 325–328.

HENSEL, G., and DURR, F. (1971), Investigations into the elimination of paraquat and its ability to be dialyzed, *Medsche Welt.*, **45**, 1791–1794.

HEYNDRICKX, A., SCHEPENS, P., and SCHEIRIS, C. (1969), Toxicological analysis of a fatal poisoning by paraquat in man, *Eur. J. Tox.*, **2**, 178–180.

IFF, H. W., BREWIS, R. A. C., MALLICK, N. P., MAWER, G. E., ORR, W. McN., and STERN, M. A. (1971), Paraquat poisonings, *Schweiz. med. Wschr.*, **101**, 84–88.

KERR, F., PATEL, A. R., SCOTT, P. D. R., and TOMPSETT, S. L. (1968), Paraquat poisoning treated by forced diuresis, *Br. med. J.*, **3**, 290–291.

KIMBROUGH, R. D., and GAINES, T. B. (1970), Toxicity of paraquat to rats and its effect on rat lungs, *Tox. appl. Pharmac.*, **17**, 679–690

LANZINGER, G., RITZ, E., FRANZ, H. E., KUHN, H. M., and KLEIN, H. (1969), Acute interstitial pulmonary fibrosis in a patient with paraquat poisoning, *Münch. med. Wschr.*, **111**, 944–949.

LLOYD, E. Ll. (1969), Recovery after taking Weedol, *Br. med. J.*, **2**, 189.

McCORD, J. M., and FRIDOVICH, I. (1969), Superoxide dismutase: an enzymatic function for erythrocuprein (Hemocuprein), *J. biol. Chem.*, **244**, 6049–6055.

McDONAGH, B. J., and MARTIN, J. (1970), Paraquat poisoning in children, *Archs Dis. Childh.*, **45**, 425–427.

McKEAN, W. I. (1968), Recovery from paraquat poisoning, *Br. med. J.*, **3**, 292.

MALONE, J. D. G., CARMODY, M., KEOGH, B., and O'DWYER, W. F. (1971), Paraquat poisoning – a review of nineteen cases, *J. Irish med. Ass.*, **64**, 59–68.

MANKTELOW, B. W. (1967), The loss of pulmonary surfactant in paraquat poisoning: a model for the study of the respiratory distress syndrome, *Br. J. exp. Path.*, **48**, 366–369.

MASTERSON, J. G., and ROCHE, W. J. (1970), Another paraquat fatality, *Br. med. J.*, **2**, 482.

MATTHEW, H. (1971), Paraquat poisoning: clinico-pathological conference, *Scott. med. J.*, **16**, 407–424.

—, LOGAN, A., WOODRUFF, M. F. A., and HEARD, B. (1968), Paraquat poisoning – lung transplantation, *Br. med. J.*, **3**, 759–763.

MICHAELIS, L., and HILL, E. S. (1933), Potentiometric studies on semiquinones, *J. Am. chem. Soc.*, **55**, 1481–1494.

MODEE, J., IVEMARK, B. I., and ROBERTSON, B. (1972), Ultrastructure of the alveolar wall in experimental paraquat poisoning, *Acta path. microbiol. Scand.*, **80**, 54–60.

MRACEK, J., and KRCH, V. (1969), Oral poisoning with herbicide 'Gramoxone', *Prakt. Lék.*, **49**, 172–173.

NAGI, A. H. (1970), Paraquat and adrenocortical necrosis, *Br. med. J.*, **2**, 669.

NIENHAUS, H., and EHRENFELD, M. (1971), Pathogenesis of lung disease in paraquat poisoning, *Beitr. path. Anat.*, **142**, 244–267.

OREOPOULOS, D. G., SOYANNWO, M. A. O., and SINNIAH, R. (1968), Acute renal failure in a case of paraquat poisoning, *Br. med. J.*, **1**, 749–750.

ROBERTSON, B., ENHORNING, G., IVEMARK, B., MALMQUIST, E., and MODEE, J. (1971), Experimental respiratory distress induced by paraquat, *J. Path.*, **103**, 239–244.

SHARP, C. W. M,, OTTOLENGHI, A., and POSNER, H. S. (1972), Correlation of paraquat toxicity, *Tox. appl. Pharmac.*, **22**, 241–251.

STYLES, J. A., and CONNING, D. M. (1969), The stimulation of fibroblastic proliferation by killed macrophages in vitro, *Proc. path. Soc. Gt Br. N. Irel.*, **67**, 10.

SWAN, A. A. B. (1969), Exposure of spray operators to paraquat, *Br. J. ind. Med.*, **26**, 322–329.

TOMPSETT, S. L. (1970), Paraquat poisoning, *Acta pharmac. tox.*, **28**, 346–358.

TONER, P. G., VETTERS, J. M., SPILG, W. G. S., and HARLAND, W. A. (1970), Fine structure of the lung lesion in a case of paraquat poisoning, *J. Path.*, **102**, 182–185.

VIJEYARATNAM, G. S., and CORRIN, B. (1971), Experimental paraquat poisoning: a histological and electron-optical study of the changes in the lung, *Ibid.*, **103**, 123–129.

VON DER HARDT, H., and CARDESA, A. (1971), Early histopathological alterations following paraquat intoxication, *Klin. Wschr.*, **49**, 544–550.

WASAN, S. M., and McELLIGOTT, T. F. (1972), An electron microscopical study of experimentally induced interstitial pulmonary fibrosis, *Am. Rev. resp. Dis.*, **105**, 276–282.

YONEYAMA, M., RAINUMA, T., and TAREVCHI, I. (1969), Swift death by poisoning caused by the new herbicide Gramoxone, *Jap. J. med. Sci. Biol.*, No. 2374, 32–34.

The Forensic Diagnosis of Acute Cyanide Poisoning

BRYAN BALLANTYNE
Ministry of Defence, Medical Divison, Chemical Defence Establishment, Porton Down, Wiltshire.

Although much has been written about cyanides and acute cyanide poisoning, the post-mortem diagnosis of poisoning by this group of compounds may not be easy. This contribution presents an approach to the forensic diagnosis of acute poisoning by cyanide, and attempts to define the problems that may be encountered. The account is limited to a discussion of poisoning by hydrogen cyanide and its salts.

A major factor in the toxic action of cyanide is the reversible inhibition of ferric iron containing enzymes. Of particular importance is the attachment of cyanide to the iron of the prosthetic group of cytochrome oxidase, resulting in a profound disturbance of the transport and utilization of oxygen in cells and causing a cytotoxic anoxia. Hydrogen cyanide, of low molecular weight and poorly ionized, diffuses rapidly and is readily absorbed through lungs, gastrointestinal tract, and skin.

The major method of detoxication of cyanide in the body is an enzymic conversion to the relatively non-toxic thiocyanate radical. Two enzymes which have been implicated in this process are rhodanese and β-mercaptopyruvate-cyanide transulphurase (Sorbo, 1962). Rhodanese (thiosulphate: cyanide sulphurtransferase, EC. 2.8.1.1), which is found principally in liver and kidney, catalyses the following reaction:

$$CN^- + S_2O_3^{--} \rightarrow CNS^- + SO_3^{--}$$

β-mercaptopyruvate-cyanide transulphurase (3-mercaptopyruvate: cyanide sulphurtransferase, EC 2.8.1.2) is present in liver, kidney, and blood, and catalyses reactions of the following type:

$$HS.CH_2.CO.COO^- + CN^- \rightarrow CNS^- + CH_3.CO.COO^-$$

High levels of thiocyanate may be encountered in the blood in cases of acute cyanide poisoning where death has been delayed: this is considered later. In addition to the formation of thiocyanate, other detoxication mechanisms include reaction with cystine to produce 2-iminothiazoline-4-carboxylic acid, and combination with hydroxocobalamin to form cyanocobalamin.

Death from cyanides has been a consequence of accidental contamination, suicidal or homicidal intent, and judicial execution. With the exception of the execution of criminals, death due to the inhalation of hydrogen cyanide has usually been due to accident, occurring particularly during fumigation procedures. In this respect it is important to remember that, since hydrogen cyanide may be readily absorbed across the skin, respirators may not give complete protection and full protective clothing should be worn (Drinker, 1932). Deaths due to the ingestion of cyanides are normally the result of suicide or homicide. The use of cyanides for suicide may be encountered more frequently in certain occupational and social groups having ready access to this group of poisons. For example, a survey of 3637 death certificates for members of the American Chemical Society revealed that of the 119 deaths due to suicide, some 35 were the result of using cyanide (Li, 1969). Occasionally, splash contamination of the eyes or skin may produce fatalities.

The estimation of what are lethal doses of cyanide to man is not easy to determine. Taken by mouth the fatal dose of hydrogen cyanide to adults is estimated at 50–100 mg., and for potassium cyanide about 150–250 mg. (DuBois and Geiling, 1959; Guatelli, 1964; Dreisbach, 1966; Camps and Cameron, 1971). Figures estimated in terms of body weight for hydrogen cyanide vary from 0·7 to 3·5 mg. per kg. (Halstrom and Moller, 1945). The effects of hydrogen cyanide by inhalation are shown in *Table* 1. By this route, the lower the concentration the greater

Table 1. Effects of various concentrations of hydrogen cyanide in the atmosphere

Atmospheric concentration of hydrogen cyanide p.p.m.	mg. per cu.m.	*Remarks*
10	11	Maximum permissible concentration
20	22	Slight symptoms after several hours
100	111	Very dangerous within 1 hour
200–400	222–444	Lethal within 30 minutes
2000	2250	Immediately lethal

is the total dose required to produce death. This is due to the fact that at high concentrations of cyanide in the atmosphere, with rapid absorption through the respiratory tract, there is a swamping of endogenous detoxification mechanisms, but when the atmospheric concentration is low the rate of detoxification may be significant in reducing the rate of accumulation of cyanide in the body.

CLINICAL MANIFESTATIONS

Although the clinical picture of acute poisoning is variable in both duration and magnitude of effects observed, the signs and symptoms may give some clues as to the cause of death. Thus the inhalation of high concentrations of hydrogen cyanide, or the ingestion of massive doses of cyanides, may produce immediate collapse with few intervening signs. In such apoplectic forms the individual may scream, loose consciousness, and fall. Sometimes a brief episode of clonic-tonic spasms may be observed. Reflexes cannot be elicited and there is mydriasis with pupillary areflexia. Breathing is sporadic and short-lived, the pulse is slow and thready, and hypotension is present. In other cases, where there has been exposure to lower concentrations of hydrogen cyanide in the atmosphere, or following the ingestion of cyanide salts, the effects may be more protracted. There may be a latent phase, following which a series of signs and symptoms are forthcoming, of which the following are the most frequently recorded.

A series of *non-specific signs and symptoms* may appear. These include headache, dizziness, constricting sensations in the chest, palpitations, weakness, nausea, vomiting, confusion, coma, and incontinence of faeces and urine (DeBush and Seidl, 1969; Hunter, 1969).

Respiratory stimulation may be observed in the early phase of poisoning. The tachypnoea and hyperpnoea observed have been ascribed to the inhibition of cytochrome oxidase in chemoreceptors, resulting in an accumulation of acid metabolites which stimulate the chemoreceptors. Direct stimulation of medullary respiratory neurones is subordinate. *Respiratory failure* follows due to depression of brain stem activity, and precedes cardiac arrest.

Effects on the *cardiovascular system* may be complex. Heart rate is often initially rapid, but during subsequent coma a bradycardia may be present which is of sinus origin or due to third-degree heart block (Wexler *et al.*, 1947; Lee-Jones *et al.*, 1970). Increased arterial pressure may be found early, but hypotension is frequently recorded later. The electrocardiogram may demonstrate an increase in T-wave amplitude, progressive shortening of the S-T segment, and eventual origin of the T-wave high on the R-wave (DeBush and Seidl, 1969; Wexler, 1947).

Convulsions often precede death. This has been attributed to anoxia of cerebrocortical neurones, although an inhibition of brain glutamate decarboxylase by cyanide has been suggested as a contributing factor (Tursky and Sajter, 1962). Inhibition of this enzyme leads to a decrease in the levels of γ-amino-butyric acid in the central nervous system accompanied by an increased tendency to convulsions.

AUTOPSY FINDINGS

Experimental observations on large mammals have demonstrated that there are no characteristic autopsy or histological appearances which allow a diagnosis of death due to acute cyanide poisoning to be made (Ballantyne, 1970). This applies to the majority of the recorded cases of poisoning in man. A variety of non-specific autopsy features have been described which are common to cyanide poisoning by all routes of administration. These include generalized congestion of the viscera, cerebral oedema, pulmonary oedema, petechial haemorrhages in brain, meninges, pleura, and pericardium (Pryce and Ross, 1963).

Some autopsy findings have been stated to be characteristic of acute cyanide poisoning. These features, together with reasons for not considering them specific, are as follows:

Odour

The characteristic almond odour of hydrogen cyanide arising from certain organs and body cavities is often stressed as important. The minimum amount of hydrogen cyanide detectable by odour is about 1·0 ppm. (Guatelli, 1964). Its presence is also detectable by the 'tobacco reaction' since, like hydrogen sulphide, hydrogen cyanide affects the taste buds in such a manner that tobacco smoke assumes an unpleasant flat metallic taste. If detectable, then the odour of hydrogen cyanide will be of obvious help but it may be missed on several occasions for the following reasons:

1. The characteristic odour may be masked by other smells such as, for example, post-mortem putrifaction. A case is recorded of a suicide who took a cocktail containing ammonia, apple juice, and cyanide. The individual was adequately treated for ammonia poisoning but died of cyanide poisoning (Camps, 1968).

2. Many individuals are unable to recognize the presence of hydrogen cyanide in the atmosphere by odour (Hunter, 1969). Various estimates suggest that between

20 and 40 per cent of the population are unable to detect a cyanide odour (Gwilt, 1961). It has been suggested that this olfactory deficiency is inherited as a sex-linked recessive (Kirk and Stenhouse, 1953), but Brown and Robinette (1967) do not believe that the inability to smell cyanide is a simple, segregating, genetically controlled trait.

3. The olfactory nerve endings are rapidly paralysed, and individuals may quickly become insensitive to the cyanide odour (Camps, 1968).

Colouration of Blood

It is frequently stated that in cases of acute cyanide poisoning the blood is bright red in colour (Simpson, 1958). This is attributed to non-dissociation of oxyhaemoglobin in capillaries as a consequence of the cytotoxic anoxia. However, observations in acute experimental cyanide poisoning (Ballantyne, 1970) and experience with human cases ha\ demonstrated that the colour of the blood may not give a clue as to the cause of death (Pryce and Ross, 1963).

Acute Haemorrhage Gastritis

Local corrosive lesions of the oesophageal and gastric mucosa may occur following the ingestion of alkali cyanide salts. The appearance is often that of a brick-coloured mucosa or intense haemorrhagic gastritis. In the absence of a characteristic cyanide odour this could be confused with the lesions of other strong alkaline poisons.

CHEMICAL ANALYSIS FOR CYANIDE

The forensic diagnosis of acute cyanide poisoning requires a quantitative analysis for cyanide to be made in blood, a variety of organs, and where appropriate on stomach contents. Only in this way is it possible to provide the surest possible foundation for eventual legal judgement.

For forensic purposes, in establishing the cause of death after circumstances suspicious of cyanide poisoning it would be ideal to establish the amount of poison taken, or administered to the victim. This, however, usually presents considerable difficulties because of the large number of factors that may influence the analytical results. These include the time elapsed between death, autopsy, and analysis; the conditions under which the corpse was kept; and the method of analysis used. Resorption coefficients have been calculated (Rusiecki *et al.*, 1960) but these can probably only be accurately applied when body tissues are obtained soon after death.

Rapid Tests for Cyanide

Several simple chemical tests have been described for the qualitative confirmation of cyanide poisoning; these have been discussed in detail by Guatelli (1964). One of the simplest qualitative tests, which may be used on gastric contents obtained by aspiration from the living patient or at autopsy, is based on the Prussian Blue reaction. A few crystals of ferrous sulphate are added to 5 ml. of gastric contents, followed by just sufficient 20 per cent sodium hydroxide to precipitate the iron. The mixture is boiled, cooled, and then acidified with 10 per cent hydrochloric acid. A green-blue colour or precipitate indicates the presence of cyanide. This reaction is not obtained with barbiturates, phenothiazines, imipramine, benzodiazepines, or amitryptaline. When salicylates and cyanide are present together there is an initial blue-green colour which then becomes masked by the purple of the ferric chloride–salicylate reaction (Lee-Jones *et al.*, 1970).

Quantitative Analysis for Cyanide

A variety of spectrophotometric and electrometric methods have been described for the quantitative determination of cyanide in body fluids and tissue homogenates. Many of these have been reviewed in detail by Guatelli (1964) and Barks and Higson (1963).

We have used a slight modification (Ballantyne *et al.*, 1972a) of the method of Feldstein and Klendshoj (1954), which is an adaptation of the technique of Epstein (1947) for use with biological materials. The technique involves separating the cyanide from biological fluids or tissue homogenates by microdiffusion or bubbling. The cyanide so separated is estimated by converting it to cyanogen chloride with chloroamine T, and reacting the cyanogen chloride with a mixture of 1-phenyl-3-methyl-2-pyrazoline-5-one and 4,4′-bis(1-phenyl-3-methyl-2-pyrazolin-5-one) in pyridine, which results in the formation of a blue dye that can be estimated spectrophotometrically at 630 nm. (*Fig.* 1).

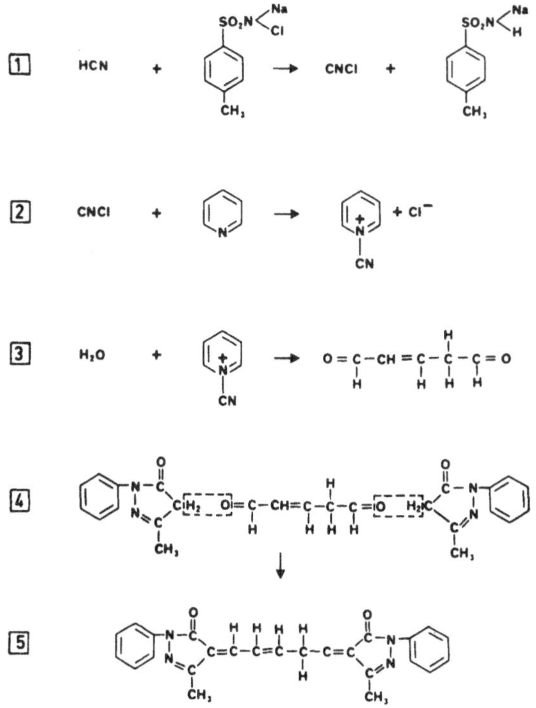

Fig. 1. Estimation of cyanide in biological fluids and tissue homogenates. The chemistry of the method is as follows: (1) Chloramine T converts cyanide to cyanogen chloride; (2) cyanogen chloride reacts with pyridine to form cyanopyridinium chloride, which undergoes hydrolysis to glutaconic aldehyde (3); (4) condensation of glutaconic aldehyde with 1-phenyl-3-methyl-2-pyrazolin-5-one to form a blue dye (5). The colour of the dye is stabilized by the presence of 4,4′-bis-(1-phenyl-3-methyl-2-pyrazolin-5-one).

Cyanide Concentrations

Although there have been many deaths as a result of cyanide poisoning, relatively few data are available on the distribution of cyanide in tissues from human fatal cases. Multiple samples from various body fluids and tissues may increase the accuracy of diagnosis and assist in defining the probable route of entry.

Typical results for the differential distribution of cyanide in small laboratory mammals killed with cyanides are shown in *Figs.* 2 and 3. The highest concentrations in such experiments are found in whole blood (Ballantyne *et al.*, 1970). It is of interest to note that when equimolar lethal amounts of hydrogen cyanide and potassium cyanide are given, then the blood concentrations are significantly higher in those given hydrogen cyanide (Ballantyne *et al.*, 1971).

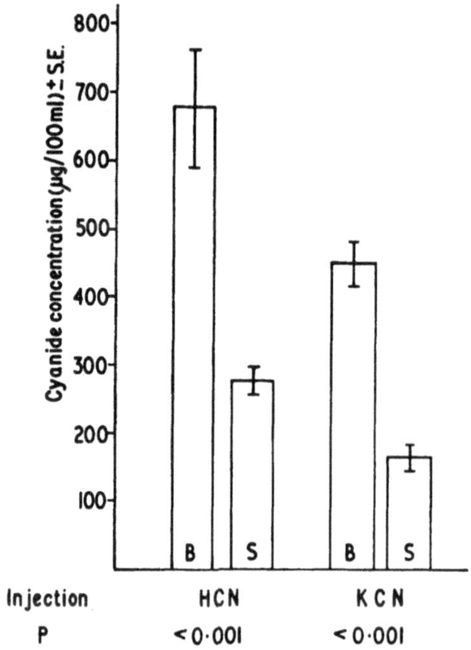

Fig. 2. Typical concentrations of cyanide in whole blood and serum following lethal intra-muscular injections of hydrogen cyanide or potassium cyanide to experimental mammals. Rabbits killed by an injection of 8 mg. CN per kg.; six animals in each group. The heights of the histogram columns represent the mean concentrations; the vertical lines are ± 1 S.E. (Data from Ballantyne *et al.*, 1972a.)

Typical values for the concentration of cyanide in body fluids and tissues encountered in fatal cyanide poisoning in man are shown in *Table* 2. The highest concentrations are found in spleen, with moderately high concentrations in blood, liver, and kidney. The concentration of cyanide in urine is low, and this fluid is not a good indicator of cyanide poisoning nor its severity. The very high levels in spleen are attributed to the binding of cyanide to erythrocytes (Sunshine and Finkle, 1964). Studies on the differential distribution of cyanide may help in assessing the most probable route of entry of poison, if this is in doubt. Thus cyanide levels in gastric contents and liver are much higher when death is due to ingestion rather than inhalation of poison.

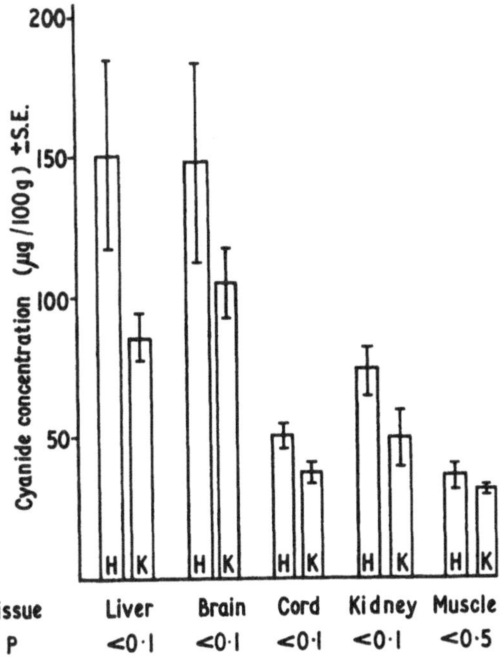

Fig. 3. Typical concentration of cyanide in various tissues from experimental mammals given intramuscular injections of hydrogen cyanide or potassium cyanide. Rabbits killed by an injection of 8 mg. CN per kg.; six animals in each group. The heights of the histogram columns represent the mean concentrations; the vertical lines are ± 1 S.E. (Data from Ballantyne *et al.*, 1972a.)

In the evaluation of cyanide concentrations, particularly when low levels are present, several factors should be taken into account of which the following are the most important:

1. Route of administration.
2. Circumstance of death.
3. Normal blood cyanide levels.
4. Post-mortem disappearance of cyanide.
5. Post-mortem production of cyanide.

Table 2. Typical concentrations of cyanide in body fluids and tissues from human fatal cases of acute cyanide poisoning*

Tissue	*Cyanide concentration (mg. cyanide per 100 ml. or 100 g.)*			
	Ingestion (34 cases)		Inhalation (3 cases)	
	Mean	Range	Mean	Range
Blood	1242	110–5310	700	100–1500
Urine	53	5–110	200	–
Spleen	4392	50–39830	–	–
Kidney	572	0–2660	110	–
Liver	773	70–2280	77	0–200
Brain	286	60–1590	140	10–340

*Calculated from cases reported by Curry (1963), Finck (1969), Klendshoj and Regent (1966), Sunshine and Finkle (1964).

Table 3. Concentrations of cyanide and thiocyanate in body fluids of normal human subjects. Results expressed as μg. of cyanide or thiocyanate radical per 100 ml.

	Cyanide			*Thiocyanate*		*Notes*	*Reference*
	Whole blood	Plasma	Urine	Serum	Urine		
Mean Range	6·4 3·5–10·1		1·0 0·1–2·5		270 110–380	Non-smokers	Maehly and Swensson (1970)
Mean Range	5·0 2·0–13·0		5·3 0·2–36		546 310–910	Smokers	Maehly and Swensson (1970)
Mean Range	4·8 0–10·7					Normal subjects	Feldstein and Klendshoj (1954)
Mean Range				146 85–265	1517 830–2000	Smokers and non-smokers	Boxer and Richards (1952)
Mean Range				220 85–265	219 78–395	Normal pregnant females	Mystrom and Sorbo (1957)
Mean Range				196 122–278		Non-smokers	Maliszewski and Bass (1955)
Mean Range				710 619–862		Smokers	Maliszewski and Bass (1955)
Mean S.E.		0·42 0·06		278 41		Non-smokers	Wilson and Matthews (1966)
Mean S.E.		0·57 0·06		667 41		Smokers	Wilson and Matthews (1966)

The effect of the *route of administration* has been briefly discussed above. In certain *circumstances of death*, cyanide may be found co-incidentally. For example, sublethal concentrations of cyanide may be detected in the blood of fire victims (Wetherell, 1966).

Published values for *normal blood cyanide levels* are not frequently seen, and those which are quoted vary because of differences in techniques, some of which do not clearly distinguish between cyanide and thiocyanate. Blood from healthy adults can contain up to 15 μg. cyanide per 100 ml. (Curry, 1969); some of the measured values cited in the literature are given in *Table* 3. The low values for cyanide in plasma determined by Wilson and Matthews (1966) may in part be due to the binding of cyanide to erythrocytes, already referred to.

Body fluids and tissues should be chemically analysed as soon as possible after their removal for two main reasons. Firstly there is a moderately rapid *in vitro* disappearance of measurable cyanide and, secondly, cyanide radical may be produced in biological tissues when they are stored for appreciable periods of time. These opposing effects, which could lead respectively to false negative and false positive results, are discussed in detail below.

Several authors have drawn attention to the *post-mortem disappearance of cyanide*, and we have quantitated this by both *in vitro* and animal experiments (Ballantyne *et al.*, 1972b; 1973). *Fig. 4* gives some idea of rate at which measurable

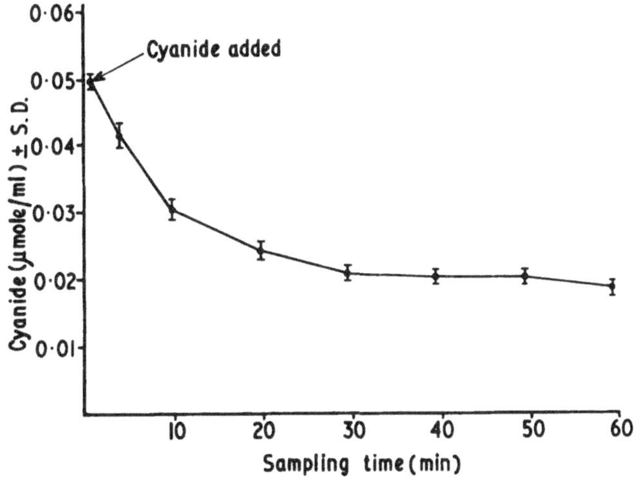

Fig. 4. *In vitro* decrease in measurable cyanide concentrations in human blood serum. At zero time a measured amount of potassium cyanide was added to a sample of serum to produce an initial concentration of 0·05 μmole CN per ml. The serum was sampled at 4, 10, 20, 30, 40, 50 and 60 minutes, and the samples analysed for cyanide. The mean of six such experiments is plotted; vertical lines represent ± 1 S.D.

cyanide may decrease in samples of serum. A few cases have been published which stress the importance of early sampling and rapid analysis to reduce this complicating factor. Curry (1963), for example, describes one case of inhalation of hydrogen cyanide where the cyanide concentration in a sample of blood taken at the moment of death was 350 mg. per 100 ml.; subsequent specimens taken at autopsy yielded a value of 50–100 mg. per 100 ml.

Various mechanisms have been advanced to explain the post-mortem disappearance of cyanide; they include the following (Ioanid and Bors, 1961; Guatelli, 1964):

1. Simple evaporation. Putrefaction accelerates the disappearance of hydrogen cyanide because of the acidic medium produced. It is essential that tissues and fluids be placed in stoppered containers to prevent escape of hydrogen cyanide, which would result in spuriously low concentrations being measured.

2. Thiocyanate formation. In the early stages this could be produced from cyanide by enzyme activity, but later transformation to alkali thiocyanate accompanies putrefaction.

$$H_2S + 2NH_3 \rightarrow S(NH_4)_2$$

$$S_X(NH_4)_2 + 2HCl \rightarrow 2NH_4Cl + SH_2 + S_{X-1}$$

$$HCN + S \rightarrow HSCN$$

$$HSCN + NH_3 \rightarrow NH_4SCN$$

3. Kiliani's reaction with aldehydes and ketones

$$R.CHO + HCN \rightarrow R.CH(OH).CN$$

Cyanohydrins are converted to α-hydroxy acids, to α-aminonitriles by ammonia and hence to α-amino acids.

4. Formation of ammonium formate.

$$HCN + H_2O \rightarrow H.CO.NH_2 + H_2O \rightarrow H.CO.ONH_4$$

5. Polymerization and transformation to aminomalononitrile

$$3HCN \rightarrow CN.CHNH_2.CN.$$

Bonnichsen and Maehly (1966) found that cyanide disappears more quickly from distillates than from the original tissue, and stress the necessity to carry out cyanide assays as soon as possible when cyanide is isolated by distillation procedures.

Post-mortem production of cyanide has been demonstrated to occur in blood, brain, liver, kidney, uterus, and the contents of stomach and intestine (Curry *et al.*, 1967). Levels which could be interpreted as being toxicologically signigicant may be produced within a few days; about 1 μg. per ml. after 2 to 3 weeks and many tens of μg. per 100 ml. after 2 to 3 months.

Patty (1921) demonstrated that *Pseudomonas pyocyanea* could produce measurable amounts of cyanide. However, Curry *et al.* (1967) found that cyanide production may occur spontaneously in bacteriologically sterile blood, and that its production was completely inhibited by the presence of 1 per cent sodium fluoride. They consider that there are at least two processes concerned – one involving the activity of certain blood enzymes, the other involving *P. pyocyanea* which appears to enhance the production of cyanide slightly. Thiocyanate oxidase may be one enzyme concerned, but it is unlikely that there is sufficient thiocyanate to account for all the cyanide formed.

Formation of cyanide occurs more readily in refrigerated samples (4°C.) than in specimens kept at laboratory temperature (Sunshine and Finkle, 1964). In the contents of the intestinal tract, post-mortem production of cyanide may occur by the slow hydrolysis of cyanogenic glycosides or other compounds containing nitrile groups. These findings underline the necessity of analysing biological material promptly after removal at autopsy. Interpretation of positive results on samples of body fluids or tissues stored in a refrigerator for a week or more requires careful evaluation.

THIOCYANATE LEVELS

In cases of acute cyanide poisoning where death has been delayed, elevated levels of blood thiocyanate are to be anticipated because of the enzymic conversion of cyanide by the mechanisms discussed previously. However, the estimation of thiocyanate in either blood or urine may not be a simple index of the amount of cyanide absorbed for several reasons. There is normally a large thiocyanate metabolic pool which fluctuates widely with variations in the dietary intake of preformed thiocyanate and plant cyanogenic glycosides (Montgomery, 1969). In addition, smokers have a higher urinary excretion of thiocyanate than non-smokers due to the intake of cyanide in tobacco smoke; the cyanide is derived from the combustion of cellulose. Furthermore, there are differences in the degree of thiocyanate excreted by smokers depending on the degree of smoking and the brands smoked (Djuric *et al.*, 1962).

Some typical values for blood and urine thiocyanate levels are shown in *Table* 3. It is difficult to give reliable limits for 'normal' levels of urinary thiocyanate. However, for the purposes of assessing the hazards to man of occupational exposure to cyanides Maehly and Swensson (1970) suggest that non-smokers who have more than 400 μg. of free thiocyanate per 100 ml. of urine should be regarded with suspicion, and likewise for smokers with more than 1 mg. thiocyanate per 100 ml.

CYTOCHROME OXIDASE LEVELS

Since the principal lethal biochemical effect of cyanide is the reversible inhibition of cytochrome oxidase, experimental investigations have been undertaken by my own group at Porton on the value of biochemical estimations for this enzyme as an aid to the diagnosis of acute cyanide poisoning. In addition, since the application of histochemical methods to forensic pathology is gaining some popularity, the biochemical estimates were supplemented with histochemical observations to define the usefulness of such techniques as confirmary tests (Ballantyne, 1972; Ballantyne *et al.*, 1972c).

Tissues were removed from rabbits shortly after dying from an intramuscular injection of hydrogen or potassium cyanide. These tissues were analysed for their cytochrome oxidase activity by the method of Pearl *et al.* (1963); typical results are shown in *Fig.* 5. Comparison of the results with those from control animals demonstrated that animals killed with hydrogen cyanide had significantly reduced cytochrome oxidase activities in all tissues examined. However, with the exception of myocardium, those killed with potassium cyanide did not have significantly different enzyme activities from the controls. This differential effect on tissue cytochrome oxidase activity may in part have been related to the generally lower tissue cyanide levels encountered in animals killed with potassium cyanide compared with those killed with equimolar amounts of hydrogen cyanide (Ballantyne *et al.*, 1972a). However, such experimental results suggest that biochemical estimations for cytochrome oxidase activity may not be reliable for confirming a diagnosis of death by acute cyanide poisoning.

Cyostat sections of similar tissues to those used for biochemistry were used for the histochemical localization of cytochrome oxidase with *N*-phenyl-*p*-phenylenediamine as substrate (Burstone, 1960). Sections of tissues from animals killed with hydrogen cyanide showed a decrease in the deposition of dye, visible under the light microscope, compared with similar tissues from controls. This was confirmed by optical desitometric measurements on the sections. However, the

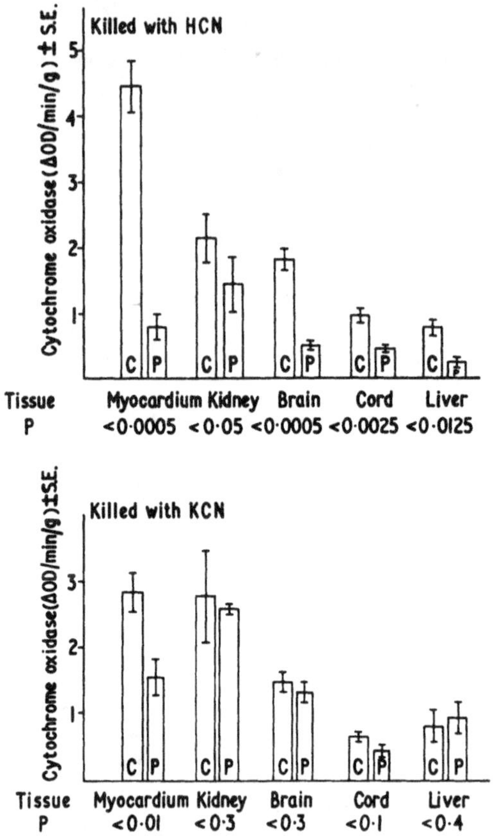

Fig. 5. Typical values for cytochrome oxidase activities in tissues from control animals and experimental animals given lethal intramuscular injections of hydrogen cyanide or potassium cyanide. Rabbits killed by an injection of 8 mg. CN per kg.; six animals in each group. The heights of the histogram columns represent mean enzyme activity, the vertical lines are ± 1 S.E. (Data from Ballantyne *et al.*, 1972c.)

inhibition was not complete, and without adequate control tissues being examined at the same time it might not have been easy to assess the histochemical reaction in terms of inhibition by cyanide. To obtain adequate controls with human preparations would be more difficult. In addition, there were no differences, either to the naked eye or on densitometry, between the deposits of dye on sections of tissues from potassium cyanide killed animals compared with tissues from controls. These histochemical findings accord with the biochemical estimates of cytochrome oxidase activity.

The above results from experimental animals suggest that a histochemical approach to the diagnosis of acute cyanide poisoning based on the demonstration of cytochrome oxidase activity is not promising as a confirmatory (or screening) test on man.

CONCLUSIONS

Poisoning by cyanides may be accidental or intentional, and can occur in the home, laboratory, agriculture, and industry. Cases of acute cyanide poisoning thus occur sporadically and unexpectedly. If the subject is seen before death, and circumstances of poisoning are not evident, then the signs and symptoms may suggest a diagnosis. The autopsy and histopathological features are not specific, and the odour of cyanide may be missed. A positive forensic diagnosis demands the demonstration of cyanide in a large number of body fluids and organs removed as soon as possible after death. Specimens for analysis should be kept in tightly stoppered containers and promptly examined. Interpretation of analytical results for cyanide requires an appreciation of the route of intake, the circumstances of death, the normal blood cyanide levels and the factors affecting these, and the knowledge that whilst there may be a rapid early decrease in the concentrations of measurable cyanide there also occurs post-mortem production of cyanide. Considerations on the differential distribution of cyanide in body tissues and fluids may assist in defining the route of intake. When death has been delayed, measurements of thiocyanate levels may help but the results require careful interpretation. Biochemical and histochemical techniques for cytochrome oxidase do not appear to be useful for confirming death as a consequence of acute cyanide poisoning.

REFERENCES

BALLANTYNE, B. (1970), Autopsy findings following death by intramuscular hydrogen cyanide: an experimental study, *Medicine Sci. Law,* **10**, 171–174.

— (1972), Experimental studies on the diagnosis of acute cyanide poisoning, *Proceedings of 4th International Meeting of Forensic Sciences,* pp. 90–91.

—, BOARDMAN, S. P., BRIGHT, J., COFFEE, D. J., WEBBER, T. D., and WILLIAMS, P. (1972c), Tissue cyanide concentrations and cytochrome oxidase activities in experimental cyanide poisoning, *Br. J. Pharmac.*, **44**, 382–383P.

—, BRIGHT, J., and WILLIAMS, P. (1972b), An experimental assessment of decreases in measurable cyanide in biological fluids, *J. Forens. Sci. Soc.*, **13**, 111–117.

—, —, — (1973), The post-mortem rate of transformation of cyanide, *Forens. Sci,* in press.

—, —, SWANSTON, D. W., and WILLIAMS, P. (1971), Toxicity of cyanides given by intramuscular injections, *Br. J. Pharmac.*, **41**, 423P.

—, —, —, — (1972a), Toxicity and distribution of cyanides given intramuscularly, *Medicine Sci. Law.*, **12**, 209–219.

—, —, and WILLIAMS, P. (1970), Levels of cyanide in whole blood and serum following lethal intramuscular injections to experimental mammals, *Ibid.*, **10**, 225–229.

BARKS, L. S., and HIGSON, H. G. (1963), A review of the methods available for the detection and determination of small amounts of cyanides, *Analyst, Lond.*, **88**, 751–760.

BONNICHSEN, R., and MAEHLY, A. C. (1966), Poisoning by volatile compounds. III. Hydrocyanic acid, *J. forens. Sci.*, **11**, 516–528.

BOXER, G. E., and RICHARDS, J. C. (1952), Determination of thiocyanate in body fluids, *Archs Biochem.*, **39**, 292–300.

BROWN, K. S., and ROBINETTE, R. R. (1967), No simple pattern of inheritance in ability to smell solutions of cyanide, *Nature, Lond.*, **215**, 406–408.

BURSTONE, M. S. (1960), Histochemical demonstration of cytochrome oxidase with new amine reagent, *J. Histochem. Cytochem.*, **8**, 63–70.

CAMPS, F. E. ed. (1968), *Gradwohl's Legal Medicine,* 2nd ed., p. 615. Bristol: Wright.

CAMPS, F. E., and CAMERON, J. M. (1971). *Practical Forensic Medicine*, p. 356. London: Hutchinson Medical.
CURRY, A. S. (1963), Cyanide poisoning, *Acta pharmac. tox.*, **20**, 291–294.
— (1969), *Poison Detection in Human Organs*, 2nd ed., p. 48 Springfield, Ill.: Thomas.
—, PRICE, D. E., and RUTTER, E. R. (1967), The production of cyanide in post-mortem material, *Acta pharmac. tox.*, **25**, 339–344.
DeBUSH, R. F., and SEIDL, L. G. (1969), Attempted suicide by cyanide, *Calif. Med.*, **110**, 394–396.
DJURIC, D., PAICEVIC, P., and KONSTANTINOVIC, I. (1961), Excretion of thiocyanate in urine of smokers, *Archs envir. Hlth.*, **5**, 18–21.
DREISBACH, R. H. (1966), *Handbook of Poisoning*, 5th ed., p. 196. Oxford: Blackwell Scientific.
DRINKER, P. (1932), Hydrocyanic acid gas poisoning by absorption through the skin, *J. ind. Hyg.*, **14**, 1–2.
DuBOIS, K. P., and GEILING, E. M. K. (1959) *Textbook of Toxicology*, p. 70. London: Oxford University Press.
EPSTEIN, J. (1947), Estimation of microquantities of cyanide, *Analyt. Chem.*, **19**, 272–274.
FELDSTEIN, M. A., and KLENDSHOJ, N. J. (1954), The determination of cyanide in biological fluids by microdiffusion analysis, *J. Lab. clin. Med.*, **44**, 166–170.
FINCK, P. A. (1969), Post-mortem distribution studies of cyanide, *Med. Ann. Distr. Columbia*, **38**, 357–358.
GUATELLI, M. A. (1964), The toxicology of cyanides, In *Methods of Forensic Science*, Volume 3 (ed. CURRY, A. S.), pp. 233–265. New York: Academic Press.
GWILT, J. R. (1961), The odour of (potassium) cyanide, *Med. leg. J.*, **24**, 98–99.
HALSTROM, F., and MOLLER, K. O. (1945), The content of cyanide in human organs from cases of poisoning with cyanide taken by mouth, *Acta pharmac. tox.*, **1**, 18–28.
HUNTER, D. (1969), *The Diseases of Occupation*, 4th ed. London: English Universities Press.
IOANID, N., and BORS, G. (1961), Contribution chimico-judiciare a l'étude des empoisonnements par l'acide cyanhydrique, *Annls Méd. lég. Crimin. Police scient.*, **41**, 275–279.
KIRK, R. L., and STENHOUSE, N. S. (1953), Ability to smell solutions of potassium cyanide, *Nature, Lond.*, **171**, 698–699.
KLENDSHOJ, N. C., and REGENT, T. A. (1966), Tissue levels of some poisoning agents less frequently encountered, *J. forens. Sci.*, **11**, 75–80.
LEE-JONES, M., BENNETT, M. A., and SHERWELL, J. M. (1970), Cyanide self-poisoning, *Br. med. J.*, **2**, 780–781.
LI, F. P. (1969), Suicide among chemists, *Archs. envir. Hlth.*, **19**, 518–520.
MAEHLY, A. C., and SWENSSON, A. (1970), Cyanide and thiocyanate levels in blood and urine of workers with low grade exposure to cyanide, *Int. Arch. Arbeitsmed.*, **27**, 195–209.
MALISZEWSKI, T. F., and BASS, D. E. (1955), 'True' and 'apparent' thiocyanate in body fluids of smokers and non-smokers, *J. appl. Physiol.*, **8**, 289–291.
MONTGOMERY, R. D. (1969), Cyanogens. In *Toxic Constituents of Plant Food-stuffs*, (ed. LIENER, I. E.), pp. 143–157. New York: Academic Press.
MYSTROM, C., and SORBO, B. (1957), Thiocyanate content of urine and blood from cases of toxaemia of pregnancy, *Scand. J. clin. Lab. Invest.*, **9**, 223–225.

PATTY, F. A. (1921), The production of hydrocyanic acid by Bacillus pyocyaneus. *J. infect. Dis.*, **29**, 73–77.

PEARL, W., CASCARANO, J., and ZWEIFACH, B. W. (1963), Microdetermination of cytochrome oxidase in rat tissues by the oxidation of N-phenyl-*p*-phenylenediamine or ascorbic acid, *J. Histochem. Cytochem.*, **11**, 102–107.

PRYCE, D. M., and ROSS, C. F. (1963), *Ross's Post-mortem Appearances*, 6th ed., p. 40. London: Oxford University Press.

RUSIECKI, W., KUBALSHI, J., and WYSOCKA, B. (1960), Cyanide content of organs in cases of fatal poisoning, *Acta Pol. pharm.*, **17**, 61–71.

SIMPSON, R. (1958), *Forensic Medicine*, p. 310. London: Edward Arnold.

SORBO, B. (1962), Enzymatic conversion of cyanide to thiocyanate, *Proceedings 1st International Pharmacological Meeting, Stockholm*, **6**, 121–127.

SUNSHINE, I., and FINKLE, B. (1964), The necessity for tissue studies in fatal cyanide poisoning, *Int. Arch. Gewerbepath. Gewerbehyg.*, **20**, 558–561.

TURSKY, T., and SAJTER, V. (1962), The influence of potassium cyanide poisoning on the γ-aminobutyric acid level in rat brain, *J. Neurochem.*, **9**, 519–523.

WETHERELL, H. R. (1966), The occurrence of cyanide in the blood of fire victims, *J. forens. Sci.*, **11**, 167–173.

WEXLER, J., WHITTENBERGER, J. L., and DUMKE, P. R. (1947), The effect of cyanide on the electrocardiogram of man, *Am. Heart. J.*, **34**, 163–173.

WILSON, J., and MATTHEWS, D. M. (1966), Metabolic inter-relationships between cyanide, thiocyanate and vitamin B_{12} in smokers and non-smokers, *Clin. Sci.*, **31**, 1–7.

Interpretation of Carbon Monoxide Levels Found at Post-mortem

D. J. BLACKMORE
R. A. F. Institute of Pathology and Tropical Medicine, Halton; attached to Home Office Central Research Establishment, Aldermaston, Berkshire★

Laboratories are frequently requested to detemine the carboxyhaemoglobin content of blood samples taken at post-mortem following the inhalation of carbon monoxide from industrial gases or car exhausts. Such analyses generally present few problems, and interpretation of the concentrations obtained are evident. In the context of accidental death associated with fire, however, the situation is more complex. Since death may be due to the combined effects of asphyxia and trauma, the subsequent interpretation of a given carboxyhaemoglobin concentration may prove problematical and require a detailed understanding of respiratory and circulatory physiology if the time interval between inhalation of the products of combustion and death is to be determined with reliability.

The final concentration of carboxyhaemoglobin in circulating blood depends upon:

1. Concentration of carbon monoxide (CO) in the inhaled gas.
2. Body weight.
3. Respiratory rate of the victim during the period over which CO is inhaled.
4. Period over which the gas is inhaled.

In a normal 70-kg. male with a cardiac output of 7 litres per minute, a respiratory minute volume of 7·5 litres, and a blood volume of 3·5 litres, the carboxyhaemoglobin (COHb) content of the blood is given by:

$$\text{COHb} = \text{concentration of CO in inhaled gas} \times \text{time of inhalation} \times 0{\cdot}5$$

In addition to the above, more obvious, parameters the results of an analysis will depend on:

1. The site from which the blood sample is taken.
2. The method of analysis.

The methods available to the analyst for the determination of carboxyhaemoglobin are numerous, but in general fall into the following three categories:

1. Spectrophotometry: these methods depend on the difference in absorption spectra of oxyhaemoglobin and carboxyhaemoglobin.
2. Protein precipitation: these techniques depend on differential thermal stability in acid solution.

★Present address: Equine Research Station, Balaton Lodge, Newmarket, Suffolk.

3. Release of carbon monoxide from carboxyhaemoglobin with subsequent measurement of the carbon monoxide –
   a. Chemically (utilizing the reducing power of carbon monoxide)
   b. Gasometrically.

Should the sample of blood be fresh, and contain only oxyhaemoglobin and carboxyhaemoglobin, then most methods are satisfactory. However, blood taken at autopsy has frequently been subjected to bacterial action and as a consequence will contain other haemoglobin pigments and volatile compounds that have reducing properties.

The use of spectrophotometric analysis is only reliable on fresh blood that has not been contaminated. Methods based on differential thermal precipitation, and comparison between a test sample and a similar sample carboxylated *in vitro* with carbon monoxide, are similarly suspect. The complete carboxylation of contaminated blood is difficult, and only by treatment of the sample with sodium dithionite and then bubbling with pure carbon monoxide for not less than thirty minutes can 100 per cent carboxylation be assured.

Techniques utilizing the reducing property of carbon monoxide following liberation of the gas from carboxyhaemoglobin are of doubtful validity in that other reducing substances will give elevated values. These methods cannot be considered to be specific.

The technique of choice is that of measuring the carbon monoxide content of the specimen by gas chromatography and comparison with the total haemoglobin concentration determined by total iron measurement and spectrophotometrically as cyanmethaemoglobin.

The interpretation of a given carboxyhaemoglobin concentration, assuming adequate methodology, will depend on the following:

1. The normal range.
2. The range following the inhalation of carbon monoxide.
3. The range experienced in fire.
4. Endogenous production of carboxyhaemoglobin.
5. Bacterial destruction of carboxyhaemoglobin.
6. Distribution of carboxyhaemoglobin following inhalation.

NORMAL RANGE

Fig. 1 shows the range of carboxyhaemoglobin detected post mortem in the victims of accidents in which there was no fire involved, and in which there was no evidence of atmospheric contamination by carbon monoxide. These are presented as a normal range because the conditions of analysis and collection are comparable to those in the remainder of this series.

INHALATION OF CARBON MONOXIDE

The simplest cases of inhalation are those in which the victims die of asphyxia following inhalation of a lethal concentration of atmospheric carbon monoxide. *Table* 1 shows the results obtained when blood samples taken at autopsy from nineteen victims of coal-gas poisoning were analysed for carboxyhaemoglobin. It is apparent that, in general, equilibration had occurred throughout the vascular

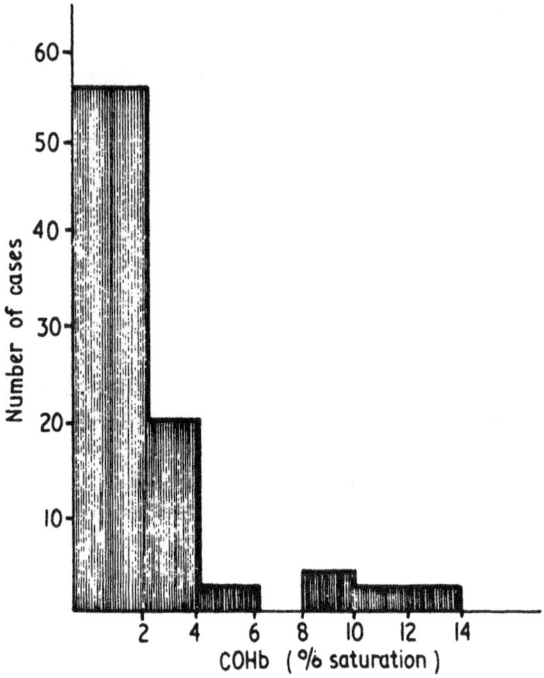

Fig. 1. Histogram showing the carboxyhaemoglobin saturation of blood taken at autopsy from 87 accident victims in which there was no fire or evidence of atmospheric contamination by carbon monoxide.

compartment; the correlation coefficients indicate that there was good agreement in individual cases.

This set of analyses were originally undertaken in an investigation concerned with the possibility that heme-containing molecules other than haemoglobin might combine with carbon monoxide during long-term exposure but not during exposure for a short period. One such heme-containing compound is the myoglobin found in muscle. Extracts of psoas muscle were analysed and found to contain much less carbon monoxide than in comparable samples of blood. In addition, there was no relationship between the amount of carbon monoxide found in extracts of muscle compared with the levels of carbon monoxide found in the corresponding samples of blood ($r = 0{\cdot}18$; slope = 0·206; $b = 37{\cdot}2$). The myoglobin was therefore separated from the haemoglobin by gel filtration and the relative concentrations of the two determined. The results indicated that the carbon monoxide present was bound solely to haemoglobin, and in spite of long term inhalation of carbon monoxide no carboxylation of myoglobin occurs *in vivo.*

Table 1. Mean carboxyhaemoglobin concentrations in blood from 19 fatal cases of coal gas poisoning.

Site of sampling	*Carboxyhaemoglobin concentration (per cent)*
Right ventricle	58·2 ($r = 0{\cdot}917$)
Left ventricle	57·8 ($r = 0{\cdot}836$)
Femoral artery	58·0
Femoral vein	61·2

Carboxyhaemoglobin determinations in accidents associated with fire is of value in assessing the period of time between physical injury and eventual death of the victim. *Fig.* 2 illustrates the general distribution of concentrations of carboxyhaemoglobin in blood from the victims of an aircraft accident in which all died at impact due to the force with which the aircraft struck the ground (incident 19/71). The

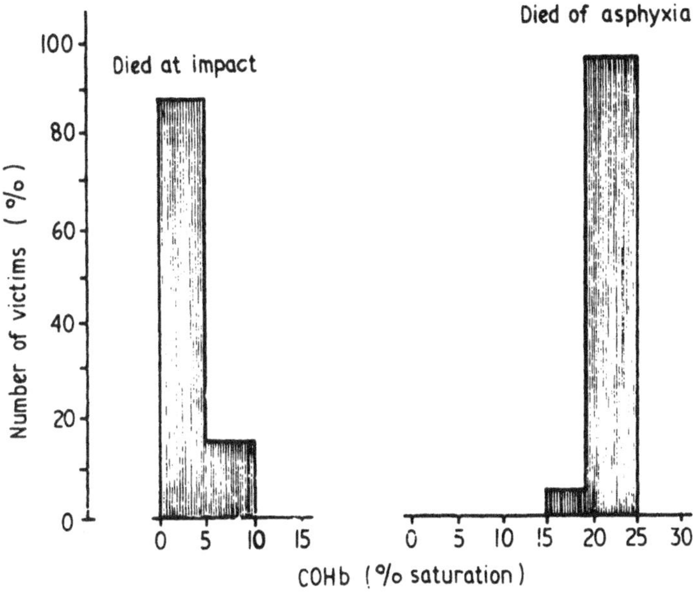

Fig. 2. Two histograms showing differences in the distribution of carboxyhaemoglobin concentrations in the victims of two aircraft accidents with differing impact forces with the ground. The histogram on the left (Incident 19/71) was constructed from carboxyhaemoglobin concentrations in the blood of victims from an accident in which all individuals died at impact. The histogram on the right (Incident 29/69) shows the distribution of carboxyhaemoglobin concentrations in blood from victims all of whom died of asphyxia in fire associated with the crash.

same diagram also shows the results from another accident in which the aircraft attempted to 'land' prior to catching fire (incident 29/69). The difference between these two histograms clearly indicates the values of such analyses in accident reconstruction. *Fig.* 3 demonstrates a mixed situation in which carboxyhaemoglobin concentrations were measured in victims of two aircraft accidents of the 'undershoot' type; half the victims died of asphyxia and the remainder died on impact.

The range of carboxyhaemoglobin concentrations found in victims of death by burning varies between 15 and 82 per cent. This wide variation emphasizes the need to examine the conditions of sampling and analysis, and to relate the results to associated pathology.

The presence of soot in the trachea is generally accepted as a good indication of the inhalation of the products of combustion, and the appearance of pulmonary fat and bone marrow emboli is indicative of the circulation of blood following burning or trauma. In a recent series of 221 victims of aircraft accidents associated with fire, 12 cases occurred in which despite soot in the trachea the carboxyhaemoglobin concentrations were less than 7 per cent. Of these twelve, five had significant pulmonary fat and bone marrow emboli indicating that in these victims not only

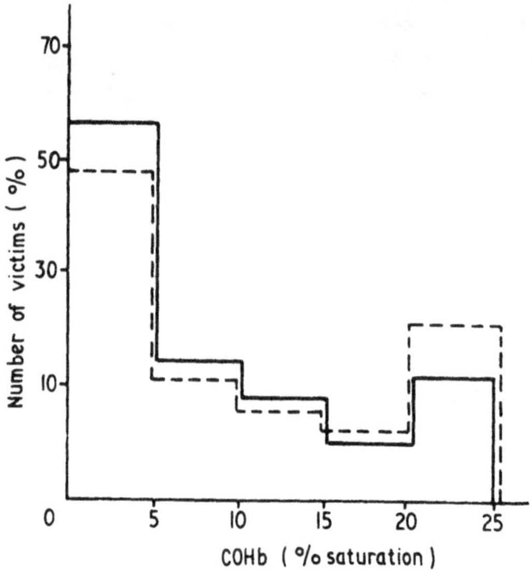

Fig. 3. Histograms demonstrating carboxyhaemoglobin concentrations in victims dying in two aircraft accidents of the 'undershoot' type. In both Incident 4/67 (continuous line) and Incident 1/69 (interrupted line) half the victims died as a result of asphyxia and the remainder on impact.

were the products of combustion inhaled but in addition blood was circulating after injury. The explanation of this apparent anomaly could be threefold:

1. Post-trauma circulation occurred prior to the fire, and death ensued before carboxylated blood in the lungs reached the heart.
2. The samples taken failed to obtain carboxylated blood.
3. The fire occurred in a well ventilated area preventing the formation of carbon monoxide.

The problems of adequate sampling are well illustrated by an incident in which the victim only survived for a few seconds following impact. The results of analyses for carboxyhaemoglobin were as follows:

Blood from pleural cavity	25 per cent COHb
Blood from right heart	16 per cent COHb
Blood from cerebellum	4 per cent COHb
Blood from aorta	6 per cent COHb

Soot was present in the trachea of this individual, and pulmonary fat emboli were demonstrated. It is clear that had only one sample been taken for analysis then a false interpretation could have been made.

OTHER FACTORS AFFECTING CARBOXYHAEMOGLOBIN CONCENTRATIONS

The inhalation of tobacco smoke will cause a rise in carboxyhaemoglobin concentration, although this rarely exceeds 8 per cent. Should such values appear significant in interpretation, then the concentration of nicotine in the urine should be determined. Typical results of such analyses are shown in *Table* 2.

Table 2. Concentrations of nicotine and cotinine in the urines of 8 aircraft accident victims in whom the presence of carboxyhaemoglobin required further explanation.

Carboxyhaemoglobin saturation of blood (per cent)	*Urinary nicotine (µg. per 100 ml.)*	*Urinary cotinine (relative amounts)*
6·7	14	+
8·0	25	+
10·0	100	+++
6·6	20	+
6·0	17	+
6·0	12	+
4·5	10	+
6·5	60	++

An incident that provided an example of carboxyhaemoglobin associated with smoking involved a Piper Comanche that crashed, killing the pilot and three passengers. The pilot and first passenger were sitting in the front of the aircraft and the second and third passengers were in the second row of seats. It was known that there was no fire after the crash, and that the four occupants of the cabin were in close proximity and would have shared a common environment until the moment of impact. The results of blood analyses for carboxyhaemoglobin and urine analyses for nicotine are shown in *Table* 3. The concentrations of nicotine in the urines of the pilot and third passenger suggested that heavy smoking and not contamination of the aircraft atmosphere with carbon monoxide was the most likely cause for the elevated carboxyhaemoglobin concentrations in their blood. The fact that these two individuals were smokers was confirmed by statements from their friends.

Table 3. Blood carboxyhaemoglobin and urinary nicotine levels in 4 individuals killed as a result of the crashing of a Piper Comanche aircraft where fire was not involved.

Victim	*Blood carboxyhaemoglobin concentration (per cent)*	*Urinary nicotine concentration (µg. per 100 ml.)*
Pilot	8	25
Passenger 1	1	0
Passenger 2	1	0
Passenger 3	10	100

Carboxyhaemoglobin is stable for many months in sterile solution when kept at 4°C. in the dark. It can, however, be denatured by bacteria to such an extent that, if estimated by a spectrophotometric technique, significant losses can occur between the time of death and the analysis of the sample. Such losses are less apparent when carbon monoxide is liberated from the sample and measured following gas chromatographic separation. Of equal importance is the production of carbon monoxide that can occur by bacteria either in the time between death and sampling, or in the sample if stored at room temperature or above. To prevent misinterpretation due to either of these effects, replicate samples from different sites should be taken at autopsy, preserved with sodium fluoride, and stored at 4°C. until analysed.

CONCLUSIONS

The interpretation of the significance of carboxyhaemoglobin concentrations determined in samples of blood taken at autopsy should not present difficulties providing that:

1. The method of sampling is adequate.
2. The method of analysis is sound.
3. The associated pathology is fully investigated.

Acknowledgements: I thank the Director General of the Royal Air Force Medical Services for permission to present this paper.

Clinical and Biochemical Effects of Lead

A. D. BEATTIE
University Department of Materia Medica, Stobhill General Hospital, Glasgow

Lead poisoning has a more ancient history than most foıms of toxicology. Paul of Aegina described lead colic in the seventh century A.D., and Hippocrates in the fifth century B.C. was familiar with its harmful effects. In modern times, important advances were made by Sir George Baker with his description of the Devonshire colic in 1767 and Henry Burton who described the blue line on the gums in 1840.

The clinical features of lead poisoning were reviewed in 50 cases by Dagg *et al.* (1965) and these are listed with their incidence in *Table* 1. Abdominal pain,

Table 1. Clinical features in 80 cases of lead poisoning*

Clinical features	*Incidence (per cent)*
Abdominal pain	90
Constipation	76
Lead line	70
Vomiting	60
Non-abdominal pain	50
Paralysis or paresis	32
Hypertension	26
Low-grade pyrexia	20
Tachycardia	18
Mental symptoms	16
Diarrhoea	12
Epilepsy	2

* After Dagg *et al.* (1965).

colicky in nature, is the most common presenting symptom and is often accompanied by vomiting and constipation. Pain and weakness in muscles especially of the thighs and shoulders may occur. Neurological symptoms are less common but a peripheral neuropathy is sometimes seen, wrist-drop and foot-drop being the initial neurological complaints in some cases. Paraesthesia can be troublesome. Psychological symptoms and even psychosis have been described and such involvement of the central nervous system can be associated with epileptic seizures.

The only specific physical sign is the Burtonian blue line which is caused by the deposition of lead sulphide at the alveolar margin. Tachycardia and hypertension have been observed in about 25 per cent of cases. A low grade pyrexia has been described in a small number of patients.

Lead poisoning frequently causes anaemia with the presence of punctate basophilic stippling and ring sideroblasts. There is a reduced erythrocyte life-span.

Renal involvement in lead poisoning may result in a nephrotic syndrome. Saturnine gout has long been recognized and raised uric acid levels with or without joint symptoms are quite frequently seen.

Lead is a cellular poison which affects many enzyme systems of the body. The effects of lead on the biosynthetic pathway of haem (shown in *Fig.* 1) are of

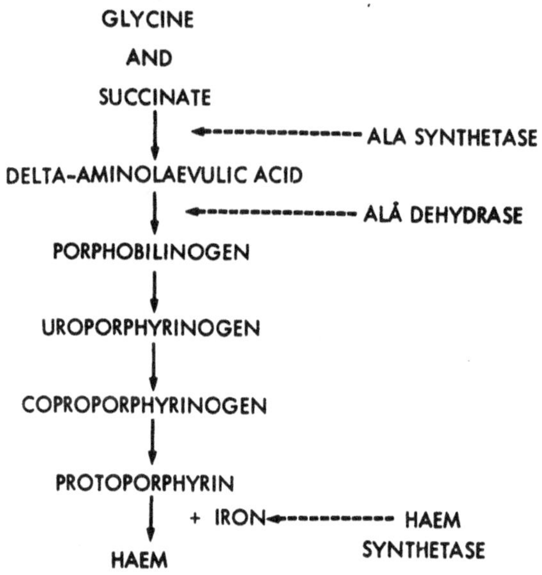

Fig. 1. The biosynthetic pathway of haem.

particular importance since the resulting abnormalities form the diagnostic tests used in lead poisoning. The enzymes delta-aminolaevulic acid synthetase (ALA synthetase), delta-aminolaevulic acid dehydrase (ALA dehydrase), and haem synthetase are known to be inhibited by lead. Other enzymes are possibly also involved and this results in increased urinary excretion of delta-aminolaevulic acid (ALA), coproporphyrin, and sometimes porphobilinogen (PBG). Protoporphyrin also accumulates and can be measured in the circulating erythrocytes.

The inhibition of ALA dehydrase is of particular interest as this enzyme is not only extremely sensitive to lead but it can be measured in the peripheral blood. *Fig.* 2 shows ALA dehydrase and blood lead in both normal and lead exposed invididuals. There is a highly significant negative correlation between the two measurements ($r = -0{\cdot}667$, $P < 0{\cdot}001$). Since ALA dehydrase falls below the normal value of 415 nmoles PBG per 10^{10} RBC per hr. when the blood lead exceeds 30 μg. per 100 g., its measurement is a very sensitive test of lead exposure.

Lead poisoning belongs to the fields of industrial and domestic toxicology and three groups are mainly at risk: the industrially exposed, children with pica and those who consume lead contaminated domestic water. There have also been occasional reports of lead poisoning from unusual sources such as lead and opium medication (Dagg *et al.*, 1965) and from the glazing of earthenware containers (Whitehead and Prior, 1960).

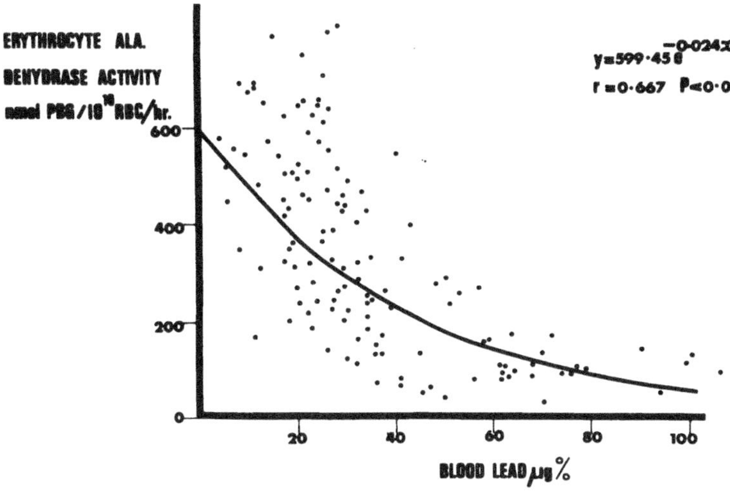

Fig. 2. The effect of lead on erythrocyte δ-aminolaevulic acid (ALA) dehydrase in humans.

INDUSTRIAL LEAD POISONING

Oxyacetylene burners form the adult group most commonly admitted to hospital with lead poisoning. Men working in shipbreaking yards are particularly at risk because of the heavy coating of leaded paint on the sections of metal being burned. The lead is vapourized by the flame and inhaled. Masks are always supplied but they tend to be worn somewhat erratically. The risk of lead poisoning is also high in scrap metal burners and smelters and in lead accumulator battery manufacturers.

The diagnosis of lead poisoning is not difficult when a patient with such an occupational history presents with abdominal pain or peripheral neuropathy. Problems arise in the protection of such workers and in distinguishing when the state of exposure to lead merges into the state of toxicity. Any worker exposed to lead dust or fumes will absorb some lead, will have a raised blood lead, and will therefore excrete lead in the urine. Not all men, however, with evidence of lead exposure are in danger of developing symptoms of lead toxicity. There is no single biochemical measurement upon which a diagnosis of lead toxicity can be based.

In an effort to evaluate the relevance of the different biochemical tests available, Gibson *et al.* (1968) studied 100 lead workers and divided them into three groups. In Group A there were 37 men without symptoms. In Group B there were 45 men with mild symptons or mild anaemia. Group C consisted of 18 men with unequivocal clinical evidence of lead poisoning including nine who were admitted to hospital. Blood lead, urinary lead, urinary ALA, urinary PBG, and urinary coproporphyrin were measured in each subject. *Fig.* 3 shows the values obtained for blood lead estimations. While the blood leads tend to be highest in Group C and lowest in Group A, there is considerable overlap between groups and there is no statistical difference between Group A and Group B or between Group B and Group C. The upper limit of normal of blood lead is generally taken to be 40 µg. per 100 g. Lane *et al.* (1968) suggest that even 80 µg. per 100 g. can be regarded as acceptable. In this study, a number of lead-poisoned workers in Group C had blood leads within the so-called 'acceptable' range. The blood lead level cannot therefore by itself be used as an absolute criterion of lead poisoning.

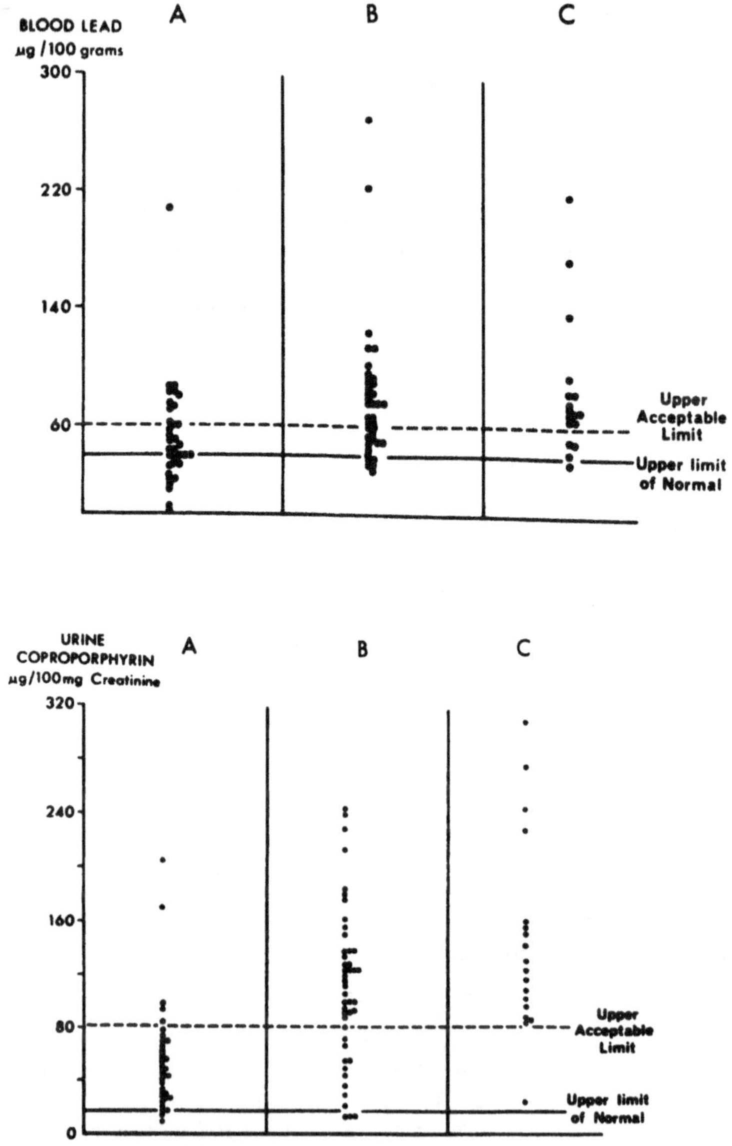

Fig. 3. Blood lead levels and urine levels of coproporphyrin, δ-aminolaevulic acid (ALA), and porphobilinogen (PBG) in three groups of industrially exposed individuals. Group A – symptom free (37 men); Group B – mild symptoms or mild anaemia (45 men); Group C – severe symptoms (18 men). (Reproduced by permission of the Editor of the *British Journal of Industrial Medicine.)*

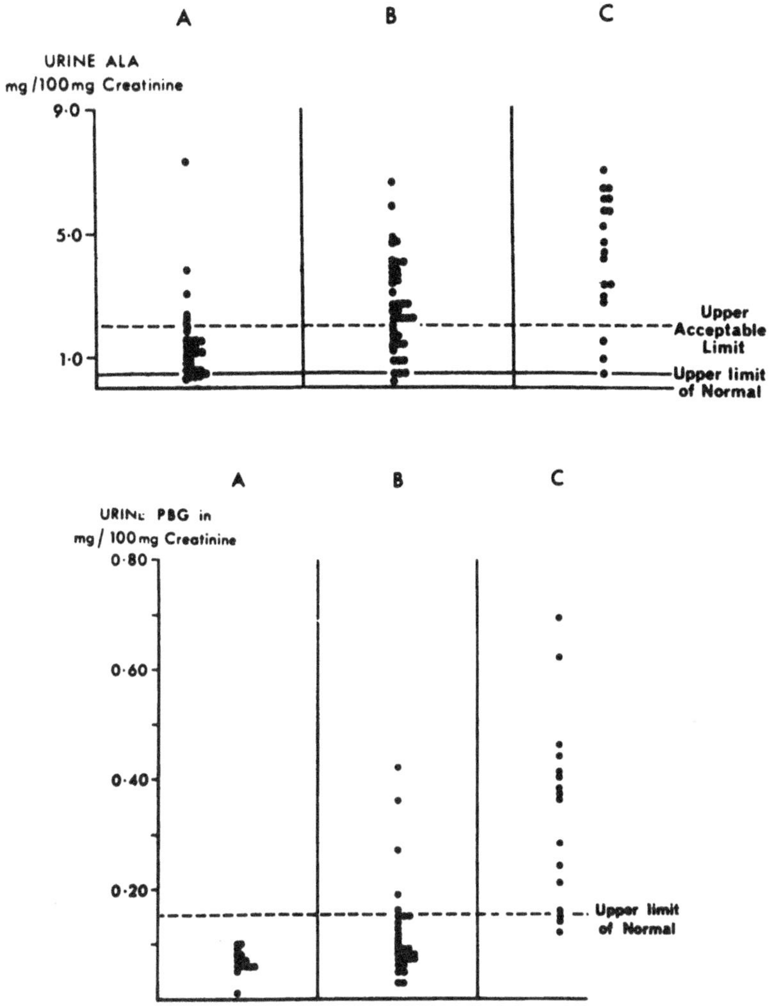

Fig. 3 (contd)

The urinary coproporphyrin results are shown in *Fig.* 3. Again there is overlap between groups but it appears that an excretion in excess of 80 μg. per 100 mg. creatinine is likely to be associated with symptoms. All groups differed significantly from each other.

The values obtained for urinary ALA excretion are shown in *Fig.* 3. Most workers with symptoms had over 2 mg. ALA per 100 mg. creatinine.

Fig. 3 also shows the urinary PBG results. The excretion of this substance was normal in all of Group A and most of Group B, whereas in most of Group C the values were above normal.

The conclusions of this study are that urinary ALA and coproporphyrin are useful indicators of clinical severity in industrial lead poisoning; blood lead is a useful, but by no means absolute, indicator; and a rise in PBG suggest severe poisoning. The overlap between groups emphasizes the absence of a single diagnostic test and the necessity to evaluate the biochemical data in conjunction with the clinical presentation of the patient.

TETRAETHYL LEAD POISONING

Rarely one may encounter poisoning with organic lead compounds, usually with tetraethyl lead – the anti-knock petrol additive. In this form of poisoning, the clinical and biochemical pattern is quite different. The subjects at risk are tank cleaners who work inside tanks which have contained leaded petrol. Organic lead fumes may be inhaled and because of the affinity of tetraethyl lead for lipids the brain is usually affected. After absorption, tetraethyl lead is converted to triethyl lead and it has been shown by Cremer (1959) that this substance is probably responsible for the toxic effects. Gastro-intestinal symptoms are not prominent and an encephalopathy occurs with insomnia, troubled dreams, anxiety, and sometimes delirium.

Four cases were recently described by Beattie *et al.* (1972a) and the principal clinical and biochemical features are shown in *Table* 2. Three patients (*Cases* 1, 2, and 4) had mild abdominal pain. One patient (*Case* 1) was admitted because of an anxiety state. Two patients (*Cases* 2 and 3) had evidence of toxic delirium which in one (*Case* 3) was sufficiently severe to make compulsory admission to a mental hospital necessary. All four patients recovered over a course of about two months.

The biochemical pattern is different in that urinary ALA and PBG were normal in all cases and urinary coproporphyrin was slightly raised in only one case. The erythrocyte protoporphyrin was moderately elevated in *Cases* 1, 2, and 3. The enzyme ALA dehydrase was greatly reduced in every case.

LEAD POISONING IN CHILDREN

In childhood lead poisoning may occur as a result of the habit of pica. This may happen where a child has access to flaking paint, especially in the outdoor situation where the lead content of paint is likely to be higher. In Britain overt lead poisoning in childhood is uncommon, although it appears to be common in the industrial areas of the U.S.A. where it may account for as many as 79 per cent of childhood deaths due to accidental poisoning (Christian *et al.*, 1964). The presenting manifestations of lead poisoning in children can be vague. Among these are irritability, vomiting, anorexia, convulsions, pallor, unsteady gait, and weight loss. Abdominal pain is less common. In severe cases, encephalopathy with convulsions and coma may occur. Pica, or an abnormal craving for substances which should not be eaten, is a common precursor of lead poisoning. Greenberg *et al.* (1958) found that, of 194 children with pica, there were 28 true cases and 20 possible cases of lead poisoning. Conversely, children who are mentally retarded are more likely to indulge in pica and Byers (1959) showed that 5 out of 45 children with lead poisoning were previously mentally defective.

Thus the most serious complication of lead poisoning in children is the possible development of mental deficiency. Perlstein and Atala in 1966 in a review of 425 surviving lead-poisoned children with a mean age of 2 years showed that 61 per cent had no sequelae, 22 per cent were mentally retarded, 20 per cent had seizures, 1 per cent had optic atrophy, and 2 per cent had cerebral palsy. Moncrieff *et al.* (1964) showed that the frequency of blood lead levels greater than 36 μg. per 100 g. in 122 mentally retarded children was 45 per cent, and Gibson *et al.* (1967) noted a higher incidence of blood lead levels greater than 40 μg. per 100 g. in a group of children with mental retardation of unknown aetiology than in normal children and mentally retarded children of known aetiology.

Table 2. Clinical and biochemical findings in four patients with tetraethyl lead poisoning*

Case	*Symptoms*	*Blood lead (μg. per 100 g.)*	*Blood ALA dehydrase (Units)*	*Erythrocyte protoporphyrin (μg. per 100 ml. RBC)*	*Urinary ALA (mg. per 24 hr.)*	*Urinary porphobilinogen (mg. per 24 hr.)*	*Urinary coproporphyrin (μg. per 24 hr.)*
1	Anxiety Insomnia Abdominal pain	80·4	74	49	4·9	2·9	117
2	Tremor Anxiety	92·5	51	73·5	2·6	2·5	188
3	Acute toxic delirium	65·7	82	64·7	3·4	1·7	293
4	Abdominal pain and shoulder pain	64·2	114	24·2	3·1	2·0	111
Normal values		<40	>400	<35	<5	<3·5	<280

*After Beattie *et al.* (1972a).

The mechanism of nervous system damage by lead is uncertain. A lead encephalopathy can be produced in suckling rats but not in adult rats, suggesting that the developing brain is more vulnerable to lead than the mature brain. The infant brain has a greater oxygen requirement and it may be that lead inhibits oxidative systems necessary for the energy supply of brain cells. Lead is known to interfere with haem enzymes which are present in every living cell including brain. ALA dehydrase which can be measured in peripheral blood has been shown to be decreased when the blood lead exceeds 30 μg. per 100 g. Millar *et al.* (1970) gave lead to lactating rats and showed a significant increase in lead content of liver, spleen, blood, and brain of the suckling rat. There was a significant and commensurate reduction in both blood and brain ALA dehydrase activity in the suckling rat (*Fig.* 4). These results suggest that even moderate elevations of blood lead may be associated with biochemical abnormalities in the developing brain.

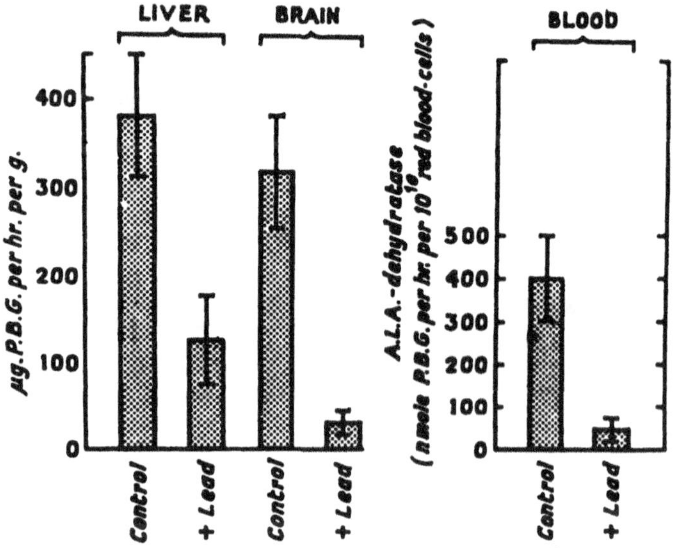

Fig. 4. δ-Aminolaevulic acid (ALA) dehydrase activity in liver, brain, and blood from normal and lead-poisoned rats.

EFFECTS OF LEAD CONTAMINATED DOMESTIC WATER

Sporadic cases of lead poisoning from lead contaminated domestic water have been described. Vitruvius referred to the unwholesome nature of water conveyed in lead pipes in 20 B.C. It was suggested by Wilson (1966) that the incidence of stillbirth or abortion in a Scottish border county might have been influenced by soft domestic water containing excessive amounts of lead. Three severe cases of lead poisoning from the Yorkshire moors were described by Bacon *et al.* (1967).

Nine people from four families living in rural parts of Scotland were found to suffer from clinical or biochemical effects of lead poisoning (Beattie *et al.*, 1972b). Five had symptoms and four had unequivocal evidence of excessive lead exposure. The source of lead was traced to the domestic water supply which in all cases was grossly contaminated with lead acquired from lead plumbing systems including lead storage tanks. The World Health Organization recommend an upper acceptable limit of lead content of 100 μg. per litre. The water lead content in the four Scottish families is shown in *Table* 3. It can be seen that in every case the source water has a very small amount of lead whereas the tap water is grossly contaminated with up to 31 times the acceptable limit.

Table 3. Lead content* of source water and cold tap water in four Scottish families†

	Source water (μg. per litre)	*Tap water (μg. per litre)*
Family 1 Sutherland	32	570
Family 2 Argyllshire	11·4	3,136
Family 3 Argyllshire	10	1,440
Family 4 Sutherland	32	1,320

*W.H.O. Limit = 100 μg. per litre.
†From Beattie *et al.* (1972b).

This study in rural Scotland provoked a similar investigation in Glasgow, which also has soft water and many houses with lead storage water tanks (Beattie *et al.*, 1972c). Twenty-three families were studied and divided into three groups according to the amount of lead in their plumbing systems. Group 1 (6 houses) had lead or lead-lined tanks for the storage of cold drinking water. Group 2 (6 houses) had no storage tank but the length of lead piping exceeded 60 ft. (18 m.). In Group 3 (11 houses) the length of lead piping was less than 60 ft. and there were no storage tanks. From each house a litre sample of overnight water was obtained for measurement of lead content and atmospheric lead was measured in a 24-hour sample from within the house. A water sample was obtained from the reservoir serving the area and its lead content measured.

Seventy-one occupants of the houses (all but two of the total) were studied. A clinical history was taken and examination performed with emphasis on the symptoms and signs associated with lead poisoning. Blood samples were taken for measurement of haemoglobin, serum urea and uric acid, blood lead and blood ALA dehydrase. Urine samples were obtained for measurement of urinary ALA and coproporphyrin and for qualitative detection of urinary protein.

The water sample from the reservoir serving the area contained 17·9 μg. per litre which was well within the W.H.O. upper acceptable limit of 100 μg. per litre. The lead content of water from the 23 houses is shown in groups in *Fig.* 5. In Group 1, the lead tank group, the mean value was 934 μg. per litre, the highest being 1850 μg. per litre. In Groups 2 and 3 the mean values were 239 μg. per litre and 108 μg. per litre respectively. There were significant differences between Group 1 and Group 2 ($P < 0{\cdot}01$) and between Group 2 and Group 3 ($P < 0{\cdot}02$).

The lead content of the atmosphere within the houses ranged from nil to 11·1 μg. per $m.^3$ with a mean of 1·46 μg. per $m.^3$ The acceptable limit for atmospheric lead content of domestic premises is 10 μg. per $m.^3$ (American Industrial Hygiene

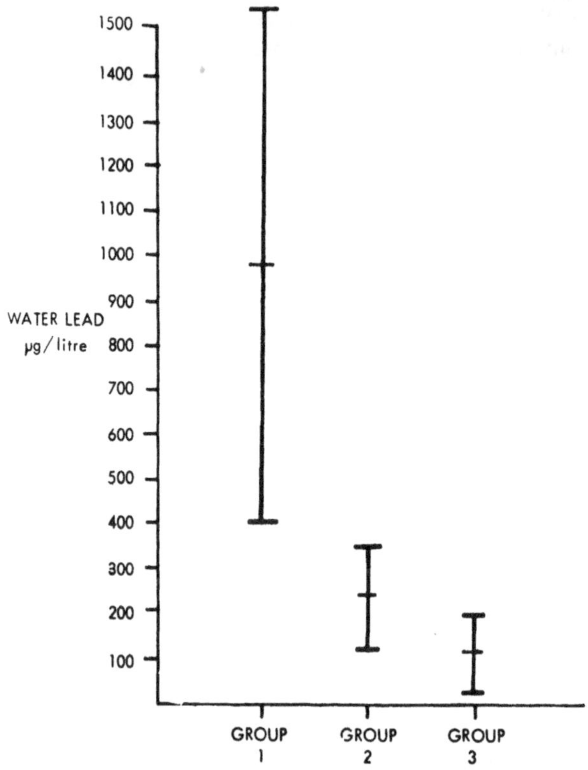

Fig. 5. Lead content (shown as mean ± standard deviation) of cold tap water in three groups with different plumbing. Group 1 – lead lined tanks for cold water; Group 2 – no tanks, more than 60 ft. of lead piping; Group 3 – no tanks, less than 60 ft. of lead piping.

Association, 1969). This level was slightly exceeded in only one house. No correlation could be found between atmosphere lead and any clinical or biochemical abnormalities. The atmospheric leads and blood leads are plotted in *Fig.* 6 and the absence of any significant correlation can be clearly seen.

Fig. 7 shows the mean and standard deviation of blood leads within each group. Three subjects in Group 1 and one in Group 2 had blood leads greater than 40 µg. per 100 g. The difference between Group 1 and Group 2 was not significant but between Group 2 and Group 3 it was significant ($P < 0{\cdot}02$). Between Group 1 and Group 3 the significance was greater ($P < 0{\cdot}001$). There was a highly significant correlation between blood leads and water leads ($r = 0{\cdot}599, P < 0{\cdot}001$).

There was a significant negative correlation between blood ALA dehydrase activity and water lead in the series as a whole ($r = -0{\cdot}535, P < 0{\cdot}001$). The mean and standard deviations within each group are shown in *Fig.* 8. Twenty-three subjects had levels below the lower limit of 415 nmoles PBG per 10^{10} RBC per hr. There were significant differences between Group 1 and Group 2 ($P < 0{\cdot}05$) and between Group 1 and Group 3 ($P < 0{\cdot}01$).

Nine subjects in Groups 1 and 2 had urinary ALA levels exceeding the upper limit of normal of 0·6 mg. per 100 ml. There were significant differences in urinary ALA excretion between Group 1 and Group 3 ($P < 0{\cdot}01$) and between Group 2 and Group 3 ($P < 0{\cdot}01$) but not between Group 1 and Group 2 (*Fig.* 9).

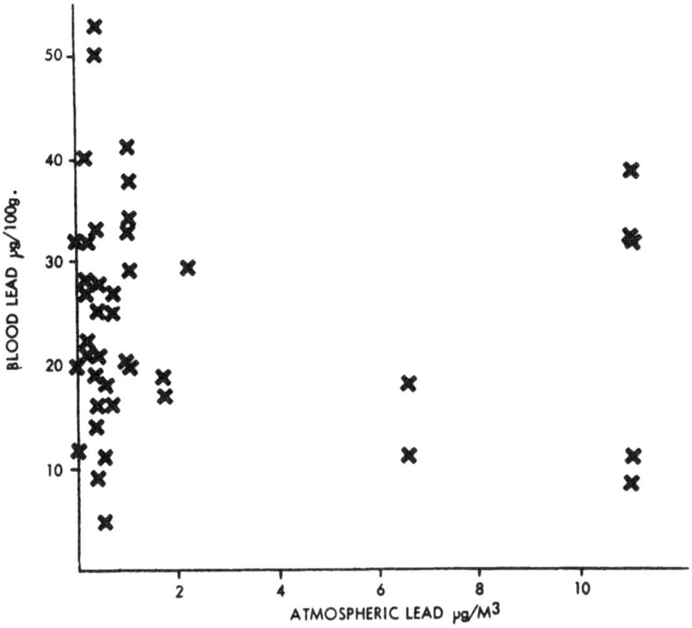

Fig. 6. Relationships between atmospheric lead levels and blood lead levels in an urban area.

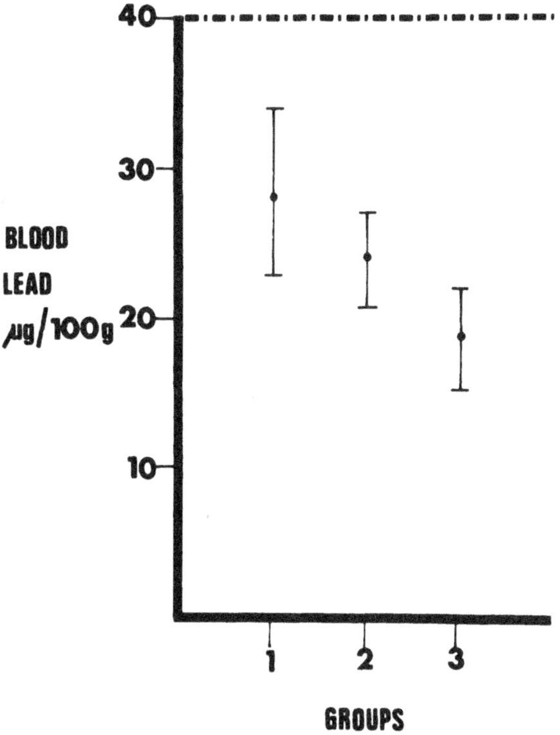

Fig. 7. Blood lead levels for the 71 individuals living in the three groups of houses shown in *Fig.* 5. Result expressed mean ± 2 standard error of mean.

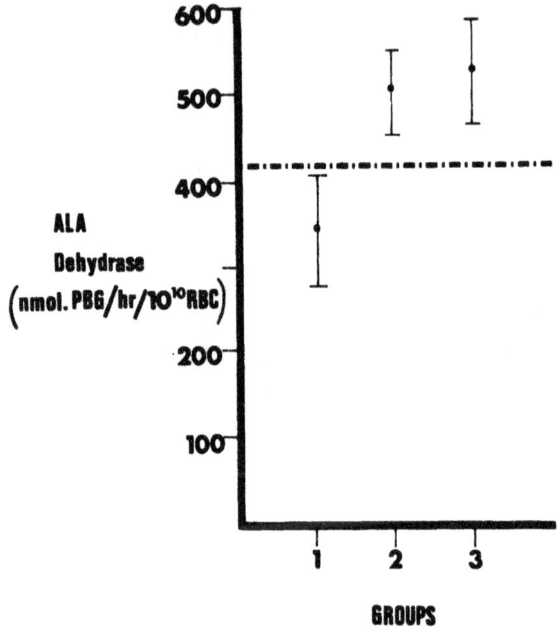

Fig. 8. Blood δ-aminolaevulic acid (ALA) dehydrase levels in the 71 individuals living in the three groups of houses shown in *Fig.* 5. Results expressed as mean ± 2 standard error of mean.

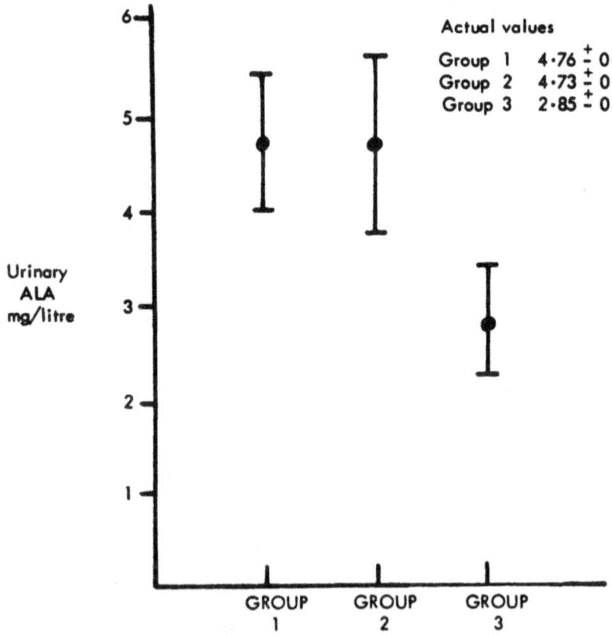

Fig. 9. Urinary δ-aminolaevulic acid (ALA) excretion in the 71 individuals living in the three groups of houses shown in *Fig.* 5. Results expressed as mean ± standard error of mean.

Urinary coproporphyrin was within the normal range in every case and levels of excretion did not differ significantly between groups. Haemoglobin, serum urea, serum uric acid, and urinary protein did not differ between groups and these measurements were not related to water lead or atmospheric lead.

A few patients complained of abdominal pain, joint symptoms, and headaches, and six were hypertensive. No correlations could be found between these clinical features and any of the biochemical abnormalities. In other words, none of the subjects had lead poisoning and the implications of the study are uncertain. It is clear, however, from the urban and rural studies, that both clinical lead poisoning and biochemical changes may result from drinking lead contaminated water.

Despite many years of research into the toxicology of lead, some major problems remain unsolved and the presence of the metal in different parts of the environment continues to endanger health.

REFERENCES

AMERICAN INDUSTRIAL HYGIENE ASSOCIATION JOURNAL (1969). **30**, 95.

BACON, A. P. C., FROOME, K., GENT, A. E., COOKE, T. K., and SOWERBY, P. (1967), Lead poisoning from drinking soft water, *Lancet*, **1**, 264–266.

BEATTIE, A. D., MOORE, M. R., and GOLDBERG, A. (1972a), Tetraethyl lead poisoning, *Ibid.*, **2**, 12–15.

—, DAGG, J. H., GOLDBERG, A., WANG, I., and RONALD, J. (1972b), Lead poisoning in rural Scotland, *Br. med. J.*, **2**, 488–491.

—, MOORE, M. R., DEVENAY, W. T., MILLER, A. R., and GOLDBERG, A. (1972c), Environmental lead pollution in an urban soft water area, *Ibid.*, **2**, 491–493.

BYERS, R. K. (1959), Lead poisoning. Review of the literature and report on 45 cases, *Paediatrics*, **23**, 585–603.

CHRISTIAN, J. R., CELEWYCZ, B. S., and ANDLEMAN, S. L. (1964), A three-year study of lead poisoning in Chicago, *Am. J. publ. Hlth.*, **54**, 1245–1251.

CREMER, J. E. (1959), Biochemical studies on the toxicity of tetraethyl lead and other organo-lead compounds, *Br. J. ind. Med.*, **16**, 191–199.

DAGG, J. H., GOLDBERG, A., LOCHHEAD, A., and SMITH, J. A. (1965), The relationship of lead poisoning to acute intermittent porphyria. *Q. J. Med.*, N.S. **34**, 163–175.

GIBSON, S. L. M., LAM, C. N., McCRAE, W. M., and GOLDBERG, A. (1967), Blood lead levels in normal and mentally deficient children, *Archs dis. Childh.*, **42**, 573–578.

—, MacKENZIE, J. C., and GOLDBERG, A. (1968), The diagnosis of industrial lead poisoning, *Br. J. ind. Med.*, **25**, 40–51.

GREENBERG, M., JACOBZINER, H., McLAUGHLIN, M., FUERST, H. T., and PELLITIERI, O. (1958), A study of pica in relation to lead poisoning, *Paediatrics*, **22**, 756–760.

LANE, R. E. *et al.*, (1968), The diagnosis of inorganic lead poisoning: a statement, *Br. med. J.*, **4**, 501.

MILLAR, J. A., BATTISTINI, V., CUMMING, R. L. C., CARSWELL, F., and GOLDBERG, A. (1970), Lead and δ-aminolaevulic acid dehydratase levels in mentally retarded children and in lead-poisoned suckling rats, *Lancet*, **2**, 695–698.

MONCRIEFF, A. A., KOUMIDES, O. P., CLAYTON, B. E., PATRICK, A. D., RENWICK, A. G. C., and ROBERTS, G. E. (1964), Lead poisoning in children, *Archs dis. Childh.*, **39**, 1–13.

PERLSTEIN, M. A., and ATTALA, R. (1966), Neurological sequelae of plumbism in children, *Clin. Paediat.*, **5**, 292–298.

WHITEHEAD, T. P., and PRIOR, A. P. (1960), Lead poisoning from home-made wine, *Lancet*, **2**, 1343–1344.

WILSON, A. T. (1966), Effect of abnormal lead content of water supplies on maternity patients, *Scott. med. J.*, **11**, 73–82.

WORLD HEALTH ORGANIZATION (1971), *International Standards for Drinking Water.*

Screening for Lead Absorption

M. H. P. SAYERS
Medical Services Division, Department of Employment

'Lead poisoning' is a term which smacks of the Poor Law and the Industrial Revolution, and I hope it will soon be deleted from the vocabulary of Occupational Medicine. It is not poisoning we should be looking for today, but evidence of undue absorption; it is with the absorption of lead that this paper is concerned.

Lead has had more than its fair share of publicity, and to maintain a sense of proportion the principal industrial hazards with which we are concerned are shown in *Table* 1.

Table 1. Principal industrial hazards investigated by the Medical Services Division of the Department of Employment during 1971

Hazard	*No. of factories visited*	*No. of workers examined*
Lead	175	5,846
Mercury	129	1,014
Cadmium	14	108
Vanadium	5	33
Fluoride	5	26
Trichloroethylene	83	617
Benzene	4	67
Methanol	2	8
MBOCA*	15	89
Organophosphates	5	53
Totals	437	7,861

*Methylene-bis-ortho-chloroaniline

Our task is to avert harm to workers from undue exposure to potential toxins. Not all hazards lend themselves to the biological approach, and in those that do, the problem is tackled in different ways. In the case of lead we can measure this in the blood. With mercury, it is simpler to examine the urine for excretion of mercury. In the case of the industrial solvents, the urine is examined for metabolites. For example, total phenol is used as evidence of undue exposure to benzene, and trichloracetic acid and trichloroethanol are used as indices of exposure to trichloroethylene (Ikeda *et al.*, 1972). A further well-tried method is to look for evidence of interference with enzymes such as cholinesterase in the assessment of exposure to organophosphorus compounds. All this can be illustrated in the context of lead.

Fig. 1 shows a simplified scheme of the biosynthesis of haem and the sites at which lead may affect the path. The excretion of δ-amino-laevulic acid (ALA) and coproporphyrin (CP) in the urine are well known indices of lead absorption, and are used by many for the screening of workers. Tests for the measurement of enzyme activity, such as erythrocyte ALA dehydratase, are not used in industry on any substantial scale as they are too sensitive for the purpose. If lead absorption is allowed to continue, then ultimately pathological effects of varying degree will ensue. Haemoglobin tends to fall, and symptoms such as lassitude and abdominal colic may result; but these are curiosities these days.

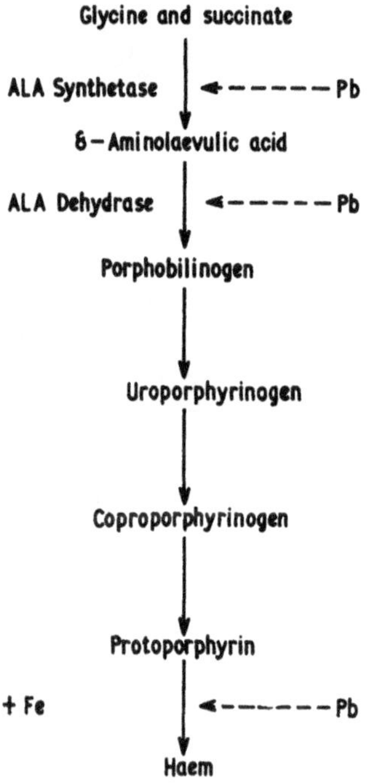

Fig. 1. The biosynthesis of haem. The sites at which lead may interfere with this pathway are shown by the interrupted arrows.

Everyone has his own favourite tests for screening lead workers, but our thinking has in recent years tended towards the identification of the degree of exposure rather than waiting for 'the response' or 'the effects'. What we need is a simple method of identifying the degree of exposure of workers engaged in a factory, and in the different processes concerned. The blood lead, of course, reflects absorption irrespective of toxic effects. At the same time it is a sensitive index of environment, more so than the conventional methods of environmental monitoring. The latter only indicate the state of affairs at a given time and place, whereas by making observations on the man we get information spread over a period of time. However, both methods have their place and are complementary to one another.

There are, of course, serious limitations to the use of the blood lead as a screening test. The difficulties of analysis and the need for venous samples have hitherto precluded its general adoption by industry in this country. There has, however, been general agreement for some years that not only medical experience but also physiological considerations warrant its use as the most satisfactory measurement of exposure. The requirement is for a simple test which is acceptable to the worker and management, and capable of being organized on a central or regional basis from a laboratory point of view. The use of capillary blood seemed to offer some promise, but the difficulties appeared considerable until this method of sampling was coupled to new developments in the use of atomic absorption spectrophotometry.

The major disadvantages of conventional atomic absorption spectrophotometry were the relatively poor sensitivity for lead, and the inefficiency of the standard nebulizer-burner systems for producing the atomic vapours. Hence, using conventional analytical methods there was a requirement for samples of large volume, necessitating venepuncture. However, recent modifications of the equipment, including the use of an atomic reservoir and tantalum boat, greatly increased the sensitivity of the method and reduced the sample volumes required to microlitres (West and Williams, 1969; Kahn and Sebestyen, 1970). A major advance which offered the best prospects of success for the use of capillary blood in determining lead levels was the introduction of a nickel microcrucible for presentation of the sample and a nickel absorption tube in the flame to concentrate the atoms (Delves, 1970). The Delves accessory is shown in *Fig.* 2.

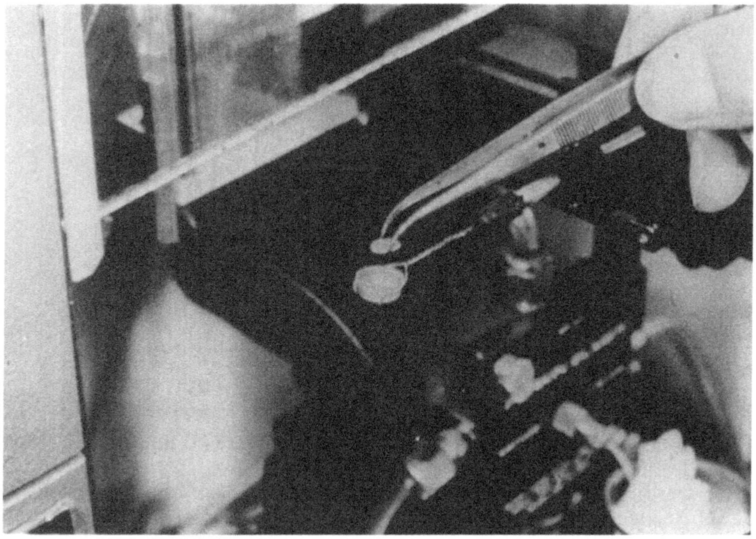

Fig. 2. The Delves microcrucible accessory for atomic absorption spectrophotometry. Using forceps, a punched filter paper disc with blood spot is placed in the crucible.

There is, of course, no question of measuring samples volumetrically in the factory, or indeed of collecting adequate samples of capillary blood by conventional methods. This prompted the idea of using alternatives, and the punched-disc technique seemed the obvious choice. Hill and Palmer (1969) have demonstrated that the results obtained from discs of blood, punched from filter paper for substances such as glucose, nitrogen, tyrosine, and urea compared in precision with those obtained after careful pipetting.

Specimens of capillary blood are collected from workers and then spotted on to filter paper and allowed to dry. Discs are punched from the spots, placed in nickel crucibles and passed into the atomic reservoir and the signal recorded. This simplifies the collection and despatch of samples, eliminates the human factor and avoids some tedious steps in analysis. *Fig.* 3 shows a typical series of absorption signals. There is good replication of the signals due to the lead (*B*) and the non-specific signals due to the combustion products of paper and blood are also seen (*A*).

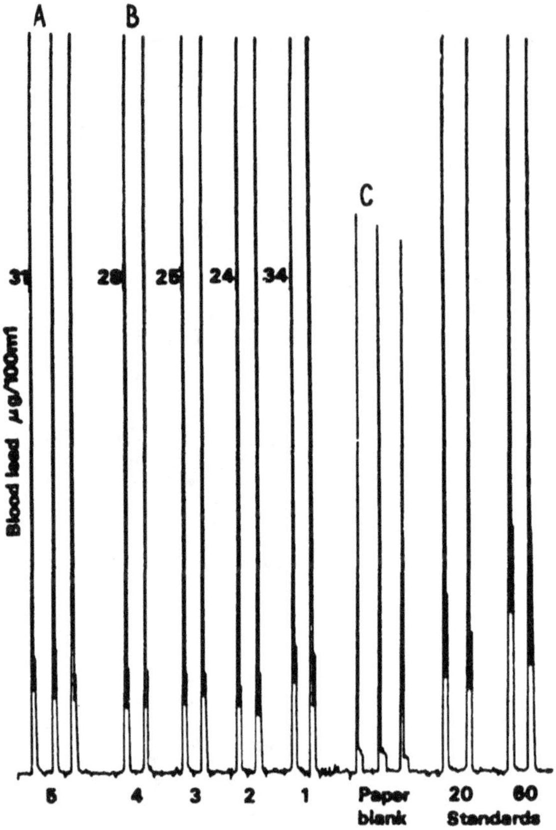

Fig. 3. Absorption signals at 283·3 nm. obtained from duplicate 6·5 mm. diameter punched discs spotted with capillary blood.
A. Non-specific absorption signal from combustion products of paper and blood.
B. Lead atomic absorption signal.
C. Signal given by blank paper and crucible.

Signals produced by the blank paper and crucible are shown separately (*C*).

Using venous samples, we estimated the lead content of blood by the micro-technique of Delves and compared the findings done by the punched disc technique. The results are shown in *Fig.* 4. Using the punched disc technique and the micro-method of Delves we then compared levels of lead in capillary and venous blood. The early results (*Fig.* 5) were sufficiently encouraging to warrant a more extensive investigation. *Fig.* 6 shows the results of the examination of 100 lead workers in 5 factories using both venous and capillary samples in each case (Cernik and Sayers, 1971). Although there was a slight negative bias against the capillary results in the lower ranges (but less than 10 µg.), the results compared well at the levels we were interested in, say over 70.

The method of collecting specimens is important. Firstly, virgin filter paper and petri dishes must be used, keeping everything covered as far as possible. Meticulous cleansing of the skin site, using a no-touch technique, is essential. The first drops of blood are allowed to run to waste as an additional precaution against contamination. A heparinized Harshaw tube is filled from the unmarked end and the appropriate piece broken off for haemoglobin estimation. The blood

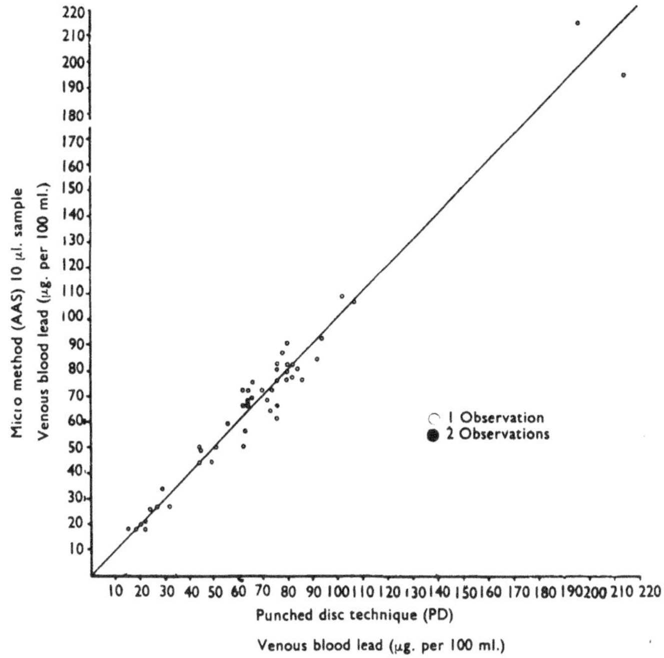

Fig. 4. Comparison of blood lead levels using the microtechnique of Delves and the punched disc technique, using venous blood.

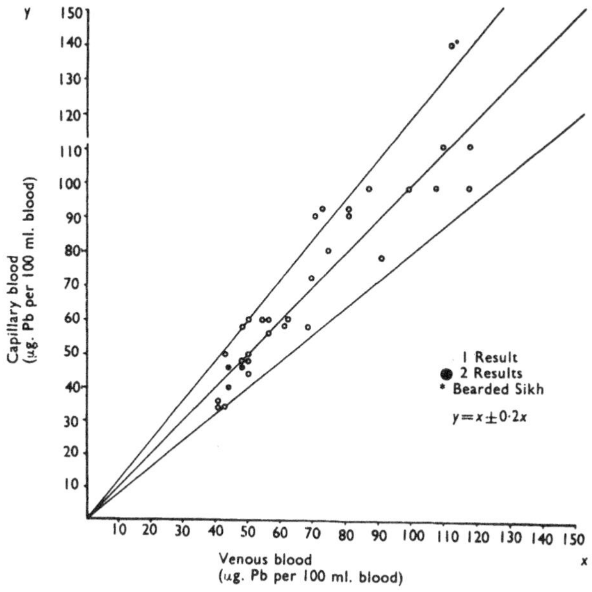

Fig. 5. First attempt to compare venous and capillary blood lead findings using the punched disc technique.

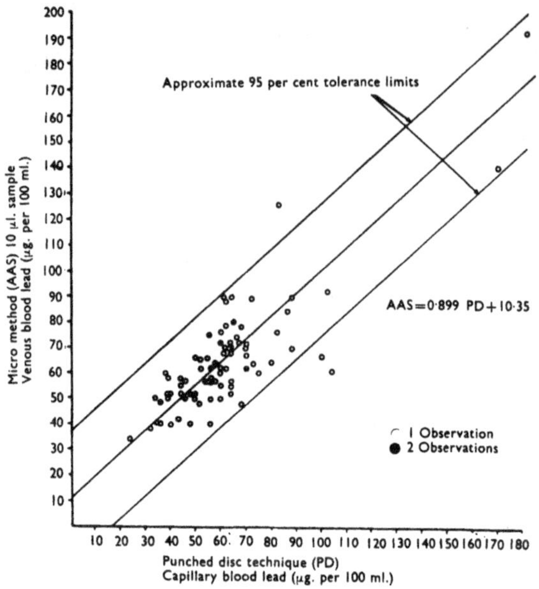

Fig. 6. The blood lead levels in 100 workers in five factories, comparing the results obtained by the punched disc technique (capillary blood) and those done by the micro-method (venous blood). The regression line and approximate 95 per cent tolerance limits are shown (Reproduced by courtesy of the Editor of the *British Journal of Industrial Medicine.*)

remaining in the tube is spotted on to filter paper (protected in a plastic petri dish) at two or more locations. The spot should be about 1 cm. in diameter. The spots are allowed to dry and the filter papers are then removed with forceps and each placed in a plastic envelope which is sealed, labelled and finally packed for dispatch to the laboratory.

The results of venous and capillary blood lead determinations in two factories are shown in *Table* 2. One was obviously a bad factory calling for the support of the industrial hygienists to advise how best to clean up the environment. Some of these workers would need suspension and medical attention. In contrast, the other

Table 2. Comparison of blood lead levels (μg. per 100 ml.) in workers at two different factories

	Bad factory		*Good factory*	
	Capillary	Venous	Capillary	Venous
	94	114	13	15
	97	84	13	20
	106	115	15	23
	115	105	17	13
	125	133	17	23
	139	123	20	21
	140	162	23	19
	150	145	23	28
	154	132	24	22
	157	115	25	23
	167	173	27	25
			33	25
Average values	131	127	21	21

was a good factory where little risk was anticipated.

On occasions, one is asked to look at men engaged in a particular process. Are they being subjected to an undue hazard and, if so, are they coming to any harm? As an example, the capillary blood lead results of one series (together with venous findings for comparison) are shown in *Table* 3. These results suggested there was obviously a lead hazard, but of low order. Even so, the industrial hygienists were called in to investigate.

Table 3. Blood lead levels in one process investigated

Serial number	*Blood lead concentration (μg. per 100 ml.) punched disc technique*		*Polarography*
	Capillary	Venous	
1	24	25	–
2	33	42	–
3	63	58	50
4	64	48	56
5	27	39	–
6	20	36	–
7	63	54	68
8	61	66	61
9	74	80	70
10	47	74	59
11	66	69	63
12	52	67	59
13	70	71	73
14	110	78	90
15	52	65	50
16	77	75	68
Group average	56	59	

The way I see the use of capillary blood lead estimations (combined with the haemoglobin) is as follows. I would stop worrying about precise figures for the blood lead as, I feel, this leads to misunderstanding. In the high risk industries – and I would emphasize this is only a personal view and not official policy – the way in which I would grade factories and workers on the basis of the mean blood lead done on capillary blood is shown in *Table* 4.

Table 4. Grading of factories and workers on the basis of blood lead levels

Blood lead (μg. per 100 ml.)	*Grade*
<50	0
50–79	1
80–120	2
>120	3

What action should be taken on such a grading system? A mean blood lead of Grade 2 or above in a factory should be regarded as an *amber light*, and is an indication to improve the environment with the help of the industrial hygienists. As for the individual worker of Grade 2 or above, reassurance is of first importance. Each man must be followed up and treated according to the results of ancillary tests. Of these, I would regard a falling haemoglobin as a *red light*, and once the haemoglobin has fallen below 12 g. per 100 ml. in a man, he should be removed from exposure. I would also regard symptoms, other than trivial ones, as a serious indication. The measurement of urinary δ-amino-laevulic acid, coproporphyrin, and porphobilinogen may assist in deciding equivocal cases. These are the minimum standards, and obviously as conditions improve we should try to raise them.

In summary, the estimation of capillary blood lead in the hands of anyone who is prepared to pay meticulous attention to detail is a useful way of supervising workers and gives an index of environment at the same time. The widespread adoption of the method, however, without realizing its inherent limitations, could be misleading owing to the real danger of contamination when taking samples in the factory. One has to bear this possibility in mind when assessing results.

We are, unfortunately, no nearer to solving the problem of lead absorption. What we have done perhaps is to help highlight it. This, we hope, will result in directing attention to the factories and processes where improvements in conditions are most needed. The ways and means of effecting this are not a medical but an engineering problem.

REFERENCES

CERNIK, A. A., and SAYERS, M. H. P. (1971), Determination of lead in capillary blood using a paper punched disc technique, *Br. J. ind. Med.*, **28**, 392–398.

DELVES, H. T. (1970), A micro-sampling method for the determination of lead in blood by atomic absorption spectrophotometry, *Analyst*, **95**, 431–438.

HILL, J. B., and PALMER, P. (1969), Filter paper blood collection and puncture as a means of quantification, *Clin. Chem.*, **15**, 381–389.

IKEDA, M., OHTSUJI, H., IMAMURA, T., and KOMOIKE, Y. (1972), Urinary excretion of total tri-chloro-compounds, trichloroethanol and trichloroacetic acid as a measure of exposure to trichloroethylene and tetrachloroethylene, *Br. J. ind. Med.*, **29**, 328–333.

KAHN, H. L., and SEBESTYEN, J. S. (1970), The determination of lead in blood and urine by atomic absorption spectrophotometry with the sampling boat system, *Atomic Absorption Newsletter*, **9**, 33–38.

WEST, T. S., and WILLIAMS, X. K. (1969), Atomic absorption and fluorescence spectroscopy with a carbon filament atom reservoir, *Analyt. chim. Acta*, **45**, 27–41.

The Comparative Toxicity of Mercury Compounds

P. LESLEY BIDSTRUP
Formerly, Department for Research in Industrial Medicine (MRC), The London Hospital

Mercury was known in the fifteenth century B.C. and its compounds used by Hippocrates for therapeutic purposes in about 400 B.C., yet the precise mode of action on biological systems remains unknown. The literature is crowded with theories as to mode of action and descriptions of experiments which demonstrate the pattern of distribution in the tissues and of excretion via the urine, faeces, lungs, and salivary glands. Man continues to react to excessive absorption of mercury and its compounds in a manner which does not change with time or theory and two types of mercury poisoning are readily distinguishable:

1. Poisoning due to inorganic mercury and its compounds such as phenyl mercury acetate;
2. Poisoning due to short-chain alkyl mercury compounds, the ethyl and methyl derivatives.

Diagnosis can be made with confidence on clinical examination provided that an adequate history is obtained, including particularly the occupational history; for today, most cases of poisoning by inorganic mercury are the result of occupational exposure and those due to short-chain organic compounds to accidental ingestion of contaminated food.

MERCURY METAL, MERCURY VAPOUR, AND THE INORGANIC COMPOUNDS

Inorganic mercury is used in many industries, the more important of which are shown in *Table* 1.

Most cases of poisoning now are due to inhalation of vapour but absorption through the skin, ingestion, or inhalation of droplets or dust of respirable particle size will also result in classical symptoms and signs of the disease. These are salivation, gingivitis, stomatitis, erethism, and tremor. Occasionally the nephrotic syndrome occurs, but this is rare, having regard to the number of persons at risk, and it is not usually accompanied by the other signs. Of these, erethism and tremor are the commonest in modern conditions of use.

Metallic mercury is heavy and therefore difficult to transfer without spilling or splashing, which results in wide distribution of multitudes of droplets tending to lodge in cracks and crevices. It is volatile at room temperature, the vapour pressure doubling with a rise of 10°F. in the ambient temperature. The large surface area resulting from spills increases the hazard considerably; thus the hazard, even when recognized, is difficult to control but it is rare in modern times to see acute

Table 1. Uses of inorganic mercury in industries and processes.

Mining and recovery from ore
Cleaning of mercury
Manufacture and maintenance of scientific instruments:
Thermometers
Barometers
Vacuum pumps
Flow meters
Mercury-cathode cell process for manufacture of chlorine
Mercury vapour turbines
Electrical industries:
Carbon brushes
Contact breakers
Switches
Rectifiers
D.C. meters
Frozen mercury casting
Fluorescent lamps and neon signs
Dry cell batteries
Manufacture of mercury compounds
Felting of fur
Finger-printing
Fermentation of beer
Amalgams:
Fire gilding
Dental fillings
Mirror making

and subacute mercury poisoning. Most cases are of mild to moderate severity arising from slow absorption over a period of months or years.

The metal when taken by mouth or injected intravenously causes few symptoms; there may be none. Injected into arteries – usually by accident in the course of scientific experiments when mercury is used as a seal in intra-arterial cannulae, or during cardiac catheterization – emboli occur in the lungs and small peripheral arteries, including those of the brain, retina, liver, spleen, mesentery, and bone. Signs of systemic poisoning may be present, also. Buxton *et al.* (1965) report nine such cases occurring as a result of cardiac catheterization.

Fatal acute poisoning of three children and serious illness of the mother is recorded by Matthes *et al.* (1958), the symptoms including cough, dyspnoea, gastrointestinal, and central nervous system effects. Death was due to acute pneumonitis. A small gas-fired space-heater had been painted with a mixture of mercury, turpentine, and aluminium which did not adhere to the surface. The heater was lit and the family retired to bed in an adjacent room. Similar effects on the respiratory system, including asthma, and on the central nervous system were common among mirror-makers in the Middle Ages (Hunter, 1955, quoting Ramazzinl).

Acute poisoning from accidental or intentional ingestion of mercuric chloride is rare now, but was a popular method of suicide in the past. Coagulation, irritation, and superficial corrosion of tissue at points of contact was followed by rapidly fatal circulatory collapse or delayed death from renal tubular necrosis. Also at necropsy, haemorrhages and ulceration were found in the large intestine.

Pink disease of infants (acrodynia) is attributed by some authorities to hypersensitivity to inorganic mercury present in antihelminthics and teething powders (Warkany and Hubbard, 1953) and a case is described in a male child, aged 6½ years, who was exposed to metallic mercury spilt on a carpeted floor from a mercury-filled bougie used by the father to dilate an oesophageal stricture (Speirs, 1959). Mercury dermatitis from mercury sulphide (cinnabar) in red areas of tattoo has been reported by Keiller and Warin (1957) and allergic contact dermatitis from the use of a mercury compound as a disinfectant in laundering by Miedler and Forbes (1968). The soluble salts, particularly mercuric chloride, are irritating to skin and mucous membranes (Sollman, 1957).

Chronic mercury poisoning of occupational origin gives rise to the curious condition of erethism, characterized by nervousness, irritability, shyness, a tendency to blush readily, and changes of temperament usually noticed first by family, friends, and workmates. Tremor follows and is usually the effect which causes the patient to seek medical advice. It is fine and rhythmical but interrupted by coarser, jerking movements. The eyelids, lips, and tongue are often affected first, the hands, arms, and legs becoming involved at a later stage. Deep tendon reflexes are present and often brisker than normal. There is no peripheral sensory loss. The nature and site of the lesion has not been identified but recent work of Fukuda (1971) confirms accumulation and retention of mercury in the brain, significantly higher in the cerebellum, the tegmentum, and the thalamus than in other structures, following exposure of rabbits to mercury vapour. A curious greyish-brown or yellow haze may be seen by slit-lamp examination of the anterior surface of the lens of the eye. It is known as mercurialentis and is an indication of exposure to mercury but not necessarily of poisoning (Locket and Nazroo, 1952).

Symptoms subside on removal from exposure and in most cases recovery is complete. It may be hastened by administration of *N*-acetyl-D-penacillamine 250 mg. q.d.s. by mouth. Hospital treatment is seldom necessary and, particularly when patients are used as 'showpieces' in clinical case demonstration, recovery may be delayed.

The clinical manifestations of poisoning, with illustrative case reports, are discussed and common occupational sources of exposure described by Bidstrup (1964). Some evidence of excessive absorption of mercury among dentists preparing amalgam fillings by hand is recorded by Joselow *et al.* (1968). Absorption through the skin may occur in the kneading of the mercury by hand and, when squeezing out excess mercury, droplets fall to the floor creating a source of vapour. Hand preparation of amalgam is being replaced by mechanical mixing in a capsule which is vibrated at high speed (5000 oscillations per minute). If the capsule is not sealed competely mercury in finely-divided form will escape. The author has seen a dental receptionist who had a relatively high excretion of mercury in the urine but no signs of mercury poisoning and who described how the 'wiggle-bug' in which the amalgam was mixed produced a film of silver dust on the glass-topped instrument tray which she wiped off with a tea-cloth or whatever else was to hand! The potential hazard of mechanical mixing, unless the capsule is sealed effectively, is considerably greater than hand preparation (Nixon, 1972). Absorption of mercury is confirmed by estimation of mercury excreted in the urine collected over a 24-hour period but a high excretion is not diagnostic of poisoning. 'Normal' output in non-exposed persons is less than 25 μg. per litre; in those at risk of absorption considerable fluctuation in mercury excretion occurs from day to day. Goldwater (1964) reports on studies of the absorption and excretion of mercury in man.

ARYL MERCURY COMPOUNDS

These have been used for many years as fungicidal and bacteriostatic agents for therapeutic purposes, as fungicides in industry and agriculture, and as slimicides in paper-pulp mills. They may irritate skin and mucous membranes, causing redness and blistering, but systemic effects rarely occur. The organo-mercurial diuretics (mainly allyl derivatives) were also used for many years, prolonging the life of many people and rarely causing symptoms which could be attributed to mercury. Thus the total condemnation of all organic mercury compounds cannot be justified.

ALKYL MERCURY COMPOUNDS

The short-chain organic mercury compounds, for example the ethyl and methyl compounds, are exceedingly toxic, causing widespread destruction in the central and peripheral nervous system. They are used mainly as seed-dressings and in bulb or potato-tuber dipping to control fungus infection. Early cases of poisoning occurred among persons engaged in the manufacture of alkyl mercury compounds; in recent times the cause has been ingestion of contaminated food.

The action on the central nervous system is selective, causing extensive but specific changes in the cerebrum, cerebellum, and long spinal tracts. There is cerebellar cortical atrophy selectively involving the granule-cell layer of the neocerebellum and the area striata of the occipital cortex. (Hunter *et al.*, 1940). Degeneration of peripheral sensory nerves occurs, the lesion ascending rapidly to the dorsal roots (Cavanagh, 1969). The resulting clinical picture is one of bizarre neurological disorder with generalized ataxia, dysarthria, and concentric constriction of the visual fields. In advanced cases disability may be total. The concentric constriction of the visual fields is due to atrophy of the area striata of the occipital cortex; the fundus oculi is normal on retinoscopy (Hunter *et al.*, 1940; Hunter and Russell, 1954).

One does not see either stomatitis or erethism in alkyl mercury poisoning unless there has been exposure also to mercury in the inorganic form, but renal failure has been reported. Höök *et al.* (1954) have described mild cases of poisoning due to short-chain organic mercury derivatives in which the symptoms were few and included unusual fatigue, impairment of memory, inability to concentrate, and numbness and tingling of the fingers with slight tremor, and Skerfving *et al.* (1970) report experiments which suggest that absorption of these compounds may cause chromosome abnormalities. They observed chromosome breakage also in persons eating fish contaminated by methyl mercury; further investigation is considered necessary to determine the significance of this finding.

Tragic episodes of alkyl mercury poisoning have occurred in recent years, due to ingestion of food contaminated by short-chain organo-mercury compounds. In 1953 an illness having all the clinical characteristics of alkyl mercury poisoning began to appear among the inhabitants, cats, and waterfowl in the vicinity of Minamata Bay, Japan. By 1970, 121 cases, 46 of which proved fatal, had occurred and a further 47, including 5 fatal, were identified at the mouth of Agano River in Niigata Province (McAlpine and Araki, 1958; Report from an Expert Group, *Nord. Hyg. Tidskr.*, 1971). The source of methyl mercury was not established until 1966 when Ui and Irukayama proved that very small amounts of mercury were produced in a process for the production of acetaldehyde by hydrogenation of acetylene where inorganic mercury is used as a catalyst. Very small amounts of methyl mercury are carried forward to the acetaldehyde distillation column and discharged with drain waste – in parts per million, diluted to parts per billion (10^9) in the main sewer. Concentrations in sea water are even lower but aquatic fauna and flora have the capacity to concentrate the organic mercury by as much as 100 times. Fish feeding on aquatic flora have high levels of methyl mercury – sufficient to cause poisoning among persons for whom fish is a principal item of diet (Ui, 1966; Irukayama, 1966). These observations, supported by the work of Jensen and Jernelöv (1969) who have shown that micro-organisms in soil and water can convert inorganic mercury to short-chain organic by methylation, have caused widespread concern about the occurrence of mercury in the environment from industrial waste and have led to the imposition of strict controls, particularly in the use of organo-mercurial fungicides, in many countries.

Jalili and Abbasi (1961) record 600 cases of alkyl mercury poisoning, many of them fatal, among persons who used grain treated with an organo-mercurial fungicide to prepare flour for home use; more recently, a similar episode of mass poisoning has been reported from Northern Iraq. When taken by mouth short-chain mercury compounds are readily absorbed and distributed to all tissues; excretion is slow.

The difference in the effects produced by inorganic mercury and the short-chain organo-mercury derivatives can be explained by differences in distribution and excretion. The aryl mercury compounds are, in this respect, similar to the inorganic compounds. Ethyl and methyl mercury compounds accumulate in higher concentrations in all tissues, particularly in the brain, and are excreted much more slowly than the inorganic or aryl compounds. Kurland (1960) found from 5 to 20 times as much mercury in the brain of persons poisoned by alkyl mercury as in those poisoned by mercuric chloride. The experimental data is recorded in detail in a Report from an Expert Group studying Methyl Mercury in Fish (1971) and a review of current knowledge is presented also.

Considerable anxiety has been generated, world-wide, concerning the possible effects of mercury contamination of food, particularly fish. Based on data obtained from Minamata, where shell-fish were found to contain 27–102 p.p.m., and Sweden, where levels of 1·7 p.p.m. for lake fish and 0·05 p.p.m. for sea fish were found, the recommended acceptable intake per day, in fish, has been set at 0·4 mg. per kg. (Expert Group, 1971). The ability of micro-organisms to methylate mercury in certain circumstances and the experience of Minamata Bay make it necessary for authorities in all countries to control disposal of mercury-contaminated waste, bearing in mind that mercury has been demonstrated in sea water, rain water, and many types of food since the early 1930s, that accurate analysis in the nanogram range is a difficult procedure, and that all forms of mercury are not equally toxic (Goldwater, 1971).

In summary the short-chain alkyl mercury compounds are highly toxic, causing irreversible damage to the central nervous system. The symptoms and signs of inorganic mercury poisoning are reversible and those of the aryl series of organo-mercury compounds relatively unimportant.

REFERENCES

BIDSTRUP, P. L. (1964), *Toxicity of Mercury and its Compounds.* Amsterdam: Elsevier.

BUXTON, J. T., HEWITT, J. C., GADSDEN, R. H., and BRADHAM, G. B. (1965), Metallic mercury embolism, *J. Am. med. Ass.*, **193**, 573–575.

CAVANAGH, J. B. (1969), Toxic substances and the nervous system, *Br. med. Bull.*, **25**, 268–273.

EXPERT GROUP (1971), Report from an Expert Group studying Methyl Mercury in Fish. *Nord. Hyg. Tidskr.*, Supplement 4.

FUKUDA, K. (1971), Metallic mercury-induced tremor in rabbits and mercury content of the central nervous system, *Br. J. ind. Med.*, **28**, 308–311.
GOLDWATER, L. J. (1964), Occupational exposure to mercury, Harben Lectures. *Jl Inst. publ. Hlth Hyg. J.*, **27**, 279–301.
— (1971), Facts about mercury, *A.M.A. Archs envir. Hlth,* **22**, 513–514.
HÖÖK, O., LUNDGREN, K-D., and SWENSSON, A. (1954), On alkyl mercury poisoning, *Acta med. scand.*, **150**, 131–137.
HUNTER, D. (1955), *The Diseases of Occupations,* p. 256. London: English Universities Press.
—, BOMFORD, R. R., and RUSSELL, D. S. (1940), Poisoning by methyl mercury compounds, *Q. Jl Med.*, **9**, 193–213.
—, and RUSSELL, D. S. (1954), Focal cerebral and cerebellar atrophy in a human subject due to organic mercury compounds, *J. Neurol. Neurosurg. Psychiat.*, **17**, 235–241.
IRUKAYAMA, K. (1966), The pollution of Minamata Bay and Minamata disease, *Advan. Water Pollut. Res. Proc. Int. Conf. 3rd.*, **3**, 153–166.
JALILI, M. A., and ABBASI, A. H. (1961), Poisoning by ethyl mercury toluene sulphonanilide, *Br. J. ind. Med.*, **18**, 303.
JENSEN, S., and JERNELOV, A. (1969), Biological methylation of mercury in aquatic organisms, *Nature, Lond.*, **223**, 753–754.
JOSELOW, M. M., GOLDWATER, L. J., ALVAREZ, A., and HERNDON, J. (1968), Absorption and excretion of mercury in man. XV. Occupational exposure among dentists, *Archs envir. Hlth,* **17**, 39–43.
KEILLER, F. E. S., and WARIN, R. P. (1957), Mercury dermatitis in tattoo, *Br. med. J.*, **1**, 687.
KURLAND, L. T. (1960), The outbreak of a neurologic disorder in Minimata, Japan, and its relationship to the ingestion of seafood contaminated by mercuric compounds, *Wld Neurol.*, **1**, 370–395.
LOCKET, S., and NAZROO, J. A. (1952), Eye changes following exposure to metallic mercury, *Lancet,* **1**, 528–530.
McALPINE, and ARAKI, (1958), Minimata disease: An unusual neurological disorder caused by contaminated fish, *Lancet,* **2**, 629–631.
MATTHES, F. T., KIRSCHNER, R., YOW, M. D., and BRENNAN, J. C. (1958), Acute poisoning associated with inhalation of mercury vapour, *Paediatrics,* **22**, 675–688.
MIEDLER, L. J., and FORBES, D. J. (1968), Allergic contact dermatitis due to metallic mercury, *A.M.A. Archs envir. Hlth,* **17**, 960–964.
NIXON, G. S. (1972), Occupational hazards in dentistry, *Community Health,* **3**, 221–225.
SKERFVING, S., HANSSON, K., and LINDSTEN, J. (1970), Chromosome breakage in humans exposed to methyl mercury through fish consumption, *A.M.A. Archs envir. Hlth,* **21**, 133–139.
SOLLMAN, T. (1957), *A Manual of Pharmacology,* 8th ed., p. 1310. Philadelphia. Saunders.
SPEIRS, A. L. (1959), Further evidence of the association between mercury and pink disease, *Br. med. J.*, **2**, 142–143.
UI, J. (1966), *Advan. Water Pollut. Res. Proc. Int. Conf. 3rd.* **3**, 167–174.
WARKANY, J., and HUBBARD, D. M. (1953), Acrodynia and mercury, *J. Pediat.*, **42**, 365–386.

The Future for Forensic Toxicology

FRANCIS E. CAMPS

I have been invited to wind-up this symposium with a discussion on the future of forensic toxicology. This is easy: at the moment it has none. To justify this remark I would add the proviso that it has no future as it is now organized and will not have until an adequate definition of forensic toxicology is reached.

At present, in some people's minds, a forensic toxicologist is an analytical chemist who, with no knowledge of physiology or pharmacology, examines autopsy specimens for drugs and poisons and often, for good measure, interprets his results. I have gone on record and will continue to assert that the behaviour of the human body when exposed to toxic substances will vary according to the nature and quantity of the substance, the manner of ingestion, and the integrity of the organs and their functions. Similarly, with infectious diseases the virulence of the invading organism and the condition of the heart will influence recovery.

I agree with Dr. A. S. Curry who has said that it is important to know the effect of the toxic substance on the cells and tissues, but in order to be able to assess this, it is essential to have a basic knowledge of physiology, anatomy, and pharmacology, not to mention pathology. With the ever-increasing complexities of analytical chemistry it is virtually impossible for a person to acquire dual qualification in chemistry and medicine and then to keep up to date.

The ultimate aim of all those who specialize in forensic toxicology must be team-work between the chemists in the forensic science laboratories and the pathologists working either in the National Health Service or in academic departments.

Without any hesitation, to my mind, the fundamental weakness of the forensic science service is the splendid mental and physical isolation from the academic and medical world which results in a dangerously narrow service. This may seem a condemnation but, to be constructive, let us consider the historical development of the service.

Until the 1930's, when Lord Trenchard established the first laboratory at Hendon, there was virtually no organization dealing with forensic science, as opposed to medicine. At that time, forensic medicine was taught in depth at some universities, especially in Scotland at Glasgow and Edinburgh, and there were adequate departments where the necessary scientific work was carried out.

In England, the analytical work was carried out by the Home Office analysts, Dr. Roche Lynch and Dr. Ryffel, both of whom had medical and scientific qualifications, or alternatively by the public analysts.

When the laboratory was established at Hendon, Lord Trenchard decided that there should be a complete and comprehensive forensic service and to this end Dr. Davidson, a well-established pathologist, was appointed as Director. To assist him were experts in analytical chemistry, biology, and serology: Dr Nichols, Dr. Walls. and Dr. Thomas. The establishment of the Hendon laboratory is well outlined by Cyril Cuthbert, who was the first liaison officer attached to the laboratory, in his book.

At that time, the coroner's post-mortem examinations were carried out by a limited number of pathologists or general practitioners; one must remember that there were few pathologists in the country then. For example, in East Anglia there were only three working clinical pathologists who were carrying out coroners' work in their spare time. Consequently, attempts were made by Dr. Davidson to obtain material in forensic medicine by obtaining access to coroners' post-mortem examinations.

This aroused the idea of competition amongst some of those who were doing the work, especially when criminal cases might be involved. This situation culminated in an argument as to who was responsible for the various ancillary examinations in criminal cases. It was eventually decided at a high level that the post-mortem examination would be carried out by the pathologist who would also do the histology, but that other examinations must be carried out in the forensic science laboratory. Consequently, for the first time, there was established a divided interest which broke up what should be perfect team-work. I do not propose to enter into the pro's and con's but it undoubtedly set back what might have been an effective service and culminated in Dr. Davidson returning to Scotland a disillusioned man; the laboratory was left without a medically qualified member of staff.

This situation still persists and that is why I say without hesitation that until this process is reversed and until the forensic science laboratories, where much of the work is done, incorporate the pathologist into their framework and their premises, forensic toxicology will make no real headway at all.

In the United States, certain chemists who work with human autopsy specimens refer to themselves as toxicologists. But what is toxicology? In the fourth edition of their book, *The Pharmacological Basis of Therapeutics,* Goodman and Gilman define toxicology as 'that aspect of pharmacology that deals with the adverse effects of drugs and is concerned not only with drugs used in therapy but also with the many other chemicals which may be responsible for household, environmental or industrial intoxication.' The toxic effects are properly considered an integral part of their total pharmacology. The toxic effects of other chemicals is such an extensive subject that the physician must usually confine his attention to the general principles applicable to the prevention, recognitition, and treatment of poisoning from any cause. But we are now dealing with many toxic substances, some with known and others with unknown toxic effects. Take, for example, the well-known story of DDT. We know that a large proportion of the population carries a burden of DDT in the body fat; Dr. C. G. Hunter and his colleagues have demonstrated this in man and also in wild-life, without apparent toxic effects being associated with its presence. We do not know what the future holds in store.

Consider another situation: if a person dies and there are negative autopsy findings, as, for example, in the Young case in Hertfordshire. The post-mortem appearances showed no pathological change to the naked eye from the point of view of poison but as a result of the police records analysis was carried out and revealed the presence of a specific toxic substance. What would the conclusion have been if it had been DDT that had been found? Would it have been assumed that the death was a consequence of DDT poisoning? In other words, *a* cause of death is not *the* cause of death; a very common fallacy in so-called forensic pathology. On the other hand, if it had been thallium or antimony that had been found, it might well be that the amounts found in the tissues represented toxic concentrations.

Here is another difficulty: unless adequate samples are taken and analysed interpretation is difficult or impossible. One often opens the newspaper to read dogmatic statements made by pathologists and coroners based on limited samples, asserting that a person has or has not died of the effects of a particular toxic substance. Then there is this wonderful term: a minimum lethal dose. There is no such thing as a minimum lethal dose: in the case of aspirin, the lethal dose may be anything between 15 and 1000 grains. The fallacy about the term is that a quantity may kill, but a person who is already ill may succumb to less than a healthy person; other factors have to be taken into account also, such as the posture and the presence of other substances, including alcohol. There is no such quantity as a minimum lethal dose.

Analysis of multiple autopsy specimens requires time, which is resented by some, and money. Results for the analysis of a single sample of blood from the peripheral circulation may not expose the truth even though eminent pathologists may express an opinion as to whether or not suicide was probable. For example, a peripheral blood barbiturate level at autopsy of 0·2 or even 0·8 mg. per 100 ml. would not be considered fatal by many but might well be if there was some postural or mechanical obstruction to respiration. The state of absorption is significant also and analysis of the liver blood and stomach contents will shed light on this aspect. These factors are important since barbiturates may either cause death due to cardiac arrest following hypotension after the rapid absorption of the drug or, alternatively, by progressive respiratory depression. Adequate analytical data together with the pathological findings will allow a proper conclusion as to the cause of death to be reached.

In my opinion team-work is a pre-requisite if the subject of forensic toxicology is to have a future.

Index

Printed in France by Amazon
Brétigny-sur-Orge, FR

51786460R00098